The Doctor-Patient Relatio

The Doctor-Patient Relationship

Paul Freeling
OBE, MB BS, FRCGP
Head, Sub-Department of General Practice,
St George's Hospital Medical School,
London, UK

Conrad M. Harris
MEd, MB ChB, FRCGP, DObstRCOG
Director, Department of General Practice,
St Mary's Hospital Medical School, London, UK

Foreword by
William A. R. Thomson
MD
Formerly Editor of *The Practitioner*

THIRD EDITION

CHURCHILL LIVINGSTONE
EDINBURGH LONDON MELBOURNE AND NEW YORK 1984

CHURCHILL LIVINGSTONE
Medical Division of Longman Group Limited

Distributed in the United States of America by
Churchill Livingstone Inc., 1560 Broadway, New York, N.Y. 10036, and by
associated companies, branches
and representatives throughout the world.

© Longman Group Limited 1967, 1976, 1984

First published 1967
Second edition 1976
Third edition 1984
First and second editions by
Kevin Browne DObstRCOG, DCH, MRCGP
and Paul Freeling

ISBN 0 443 02375 1

British Library Cataloguing in Publication Data
Freeling, Paul
    The doctor-patient relationship.
    1. Physician and patient
    I. Title   II. Harris, C.
    610.69′6   R727.3

Library of Congress Cataloguing in Publication Data
Freeling, Paul.
    The doctor-patient relationship.

    Rev. ed. of: The doctor-patient relationship/
Kevin Browne, Paul Freeling. 2nd ed. 1976.
    1. Physician and patient. I. Harris, Conrad M.
(Conrad Michael) II. Browne, Kevin. Doctor-patient
relationship. III. Title. [DNLM: 1. Physician-Patient
relations. W 62 F854d]
R727.3.F67   1984   610.69′6   83–2046

Printed in Singapore by Selector Printing Co Pte Ltd.

Foreword to the First Edition

By William A. R. Thomson MD
Formerly Editor of *The Practitioner*

The doctor-patient relationship is the basis of good general practice. This truism, which has tended to be submerged during the last two decades of medico-political controversy and increasing specialisation, is now being re-recognised. Whilst lip-service has been paid to its importance by specialists, politicians and ex cathedra commentators, those general practitioners brought up in the tradition of the family doctor have been carrying precept into practice.

In this book, which consists of a series of articles published in *The Practitioner* throughout 1966, two partners in general practice explain precisely what is meant by the doctor-patient relationship, illustrating their teaching with a series of case histories from their own practice. This is no mere academic exercise. It is teaching based entirely on experience and the hard facts of life.

But it not only provides the facts which the prospective general practitioner needs if he is to make a success of his career, it provides abundant evidence that, in the words of the authors, 'satisfactions to be obtained from general practice are probably greater than from any other branch of medicine. They are to be found in the exercising of the general practitioner's special function and not in the imitation of the specialist. ... If diagnosis were easy and treatment difficult the general practitioner's role would be degraded to a menial task, but the reverse is true. In many major illnesses nowadays the initial diagnosis is the one difficult discipline. Once the decision for hospital admission is made the sequel is usually a matter of routine, much, if not all, of which can be handled by junior staff or technicians.'

In making this 'initial diagnosis' the doctor-patient relationship often plays a crucial part, and in explaining in precise terms exactly what this relationship involves, how it can be cultivated and how it works in practice the authors of this book have been brilliantly successful.

This is no idle claim, but a statement based upon the many complimentary letters received from readers and the steady stream of requests from readers all over the world, in the first place for reprints of the articles as they appeared, and subsequently for their republication in book form. This is a book that will appeal to every general practitioner. Even the most experienced will learn something from its pages, whilst the younger generation will find it an invaluable guide to the intricacies of general practice.

5 Bentinck Street, London W1
January 1967

Preface to the Third Edition

The first edition of this book was published in 1967; it consisted of a series of articles published in *The Practitioner* in 1966 and was written for established general practitioners. Dr William A. R. Thompson said in his foreword that its authors set out to 'explain precisely what is meant by the doctor-patient relationship, illustrating their teaching with a series of case-histories from their own practice. This is no mere academic exercise—it is teaching based entirely on experience and the hard facts of the case.'

A second edition appeared in 1975. It contained additions which reflected the changes that had taken place in the attitudes of the medical profession, and tried particularly to meet the needs of general practitioner trainers.

Kevin Browne has now retired from general practice, and this third edition has a new co-author. It has been extensively re-written in the light of further experience and of the work of many people who have studied the subject in many ways. We believe that the original approach remains valid, and we hope that the inclusion of so many case-histories of our own patients will make the book useful both to everyone working in the arena of general practice—medical students, trainers and established practitioners—and to non-medical readers interested in understanding a relationship in which they have every chance of becoming involved.

We would like to acknowledge the debts we owe to Sheila Skipp for typing the manuscript, helped by Frances Hanson and Moira Jenkins, and to all our patients who made us think.

London, 1983   P. F.
                                                         C. M. H.

A process cannot be understood by stopping it. Understanding must move with the flow of the process, must join it and flow with it.

First Law of Mentat
Frank Herbert

Contents

1

An introduction

General practice in the United Kingdom passed through a phase of depression (the '50s) and a phase of euphoria (the late '60s) before reaching a phase of sanguine responsibility (the late '70s). General practitioners teach medical students and, at last, a few pre-registration housemen; they train would-be principals and seek responsibility for their own continuing education. In other countries there has been a similar revival of general practice, and in the United States of America it has been resurrected as Family Medicine. In the 1980s general practice will expand its research into its own functions and organisation, and fulfil its fundamental role with an increasing emphasis on preventive and anticipatory care.

As general practice adopts the dignity and responsibilities of a discrete discipline, with ever-widening horizons, the special function of its practitioners remains unchanged, and it is from this that all else stems. The special function is to accept any presentation of malaise that a patient chooses to make and to assess it before intervening. This demands that the general practitioner understand as much as possible of his patients' communications.

In meeting its newer responsibilities general practice has increased the complexity of its organisation, placing hurdles rather than an open door between practitioner and patient; it has adopted notions of teamwork and delegation that threaten the reality of a continuing, personal doctor-patient relationship. The claim of general practice to provide 'whole-person' care is now made by other disciplines and the meaning of the term has become blurred by its general acceptance.

> Twenty-year-old Mrs Avis, with severe facial scarring from persisting acne, was referred to a dermatologist with the specific question 'Is planing of this girl's skin feasible?' The general practitioner had described all her problems, including her massive social difficulties and the sense of stigma which made it more difficult for her to manage them. He had also stated that he would continue to see Mrs Avis himself. Several out-patient visits later, her skin was worse rather than better, after only slight variations on treatment the general

practitioner had already prescribed. In addition, Mrs Avis was now taking twice daily phenobarbitone. She did not see why she needed this and said that it hindered her ability to cope.

The dermatological registrar telephoned the general practitioner : 'We can't treat just Mrs Avis's face; we must treat her as a whole person.' The general practitioner wondered for a moment whether he had been acting selfishly in his relationship with Mrs Avis to his patient's disadvantage. 'How will you treat her as a whole person?' he asked. 'We would like to admit her to our wards and have our social worker see her,' replied the registrar.

It is no less possible today than it has ever been for the general practitioner, like Mrs Avis's dermatological registrar, to fly from the realities he perceives in his relationship with the patient. He can use the team of colleagues with which, in the United Kingdom at least, he has been provided. He can add yet another item to the inexorable increase in prescriptions for psychotropic drugs. No direct criticism of the team approach is made or implied, nor any claim that the general practitioner must always be its leader. It is not implied that drug treatment is wrong, or that delegation of care to others is inappropriate. We simply insist that all actions taken by a general practitioner with and for a patient affect him, the patient and their relationship. He must infer from the relationship how the patient will react to what he does, and what effects this will have.

The first-contact role

The person to whom a patient first turns for professional help is being offered a specific and emotionally important role. It is easy to delegate professional tasks, but this 'first-contact' role cannot be delegated—at least not without an investment of time, skill and concern which might be better deployed in helping the patient directly.

'All problem' care

The general practitioner must be careful to avoid using the psychological and social problems which he elicits simply as two new categories of 'disease' to be added to those by which patients can be distributed to new specialists like social workers, clinical psychologists or community psychiatric nurses. Perhaps 'all-problem' care would have been a more sensible term than 'whole-person' care.

Mrs Bellamy, a new patient, brought her baby Kerry to the doctor. She was plain and drab; the baby was as pretty and bright as a doll. Mrs Bellamy complained that Kerry had another cold and was coughing again. As she undressed the baby, the doctor saw that Kerry had ectopy of the bladder and that Mrs Bellamy was steadfastly looking the other way, handling the undressed baby efficiently but with some distaste. The child was laughing and gurgling, plump and happy, with no signs of any respiratory infection. 'What am I going to do about all these colds? I get worried about Kerry. I just sit and cry sometimes. My other doctor gave me some tablets for my depression but they didn't help so I stopped them.'

The doctor prompted Mrs Bellamy to tell him a little more about herself. She had married her husband, who was 20 years older than herself, five years earlier. After a year without falling pregnant she had been investigated for infertility; no abnormality had been discovered and she had conceived after a further two and a half years. A relatively easy pregnancy and labour had resulted in the birth of Kerry. 'I do so want another baby and I had such trouble falling for Kerry,' she concluded, still looking drab, depressed and frozen-faced.

The doctor reflected that some depression was common enough in a mother with a baby of Kerry's age, all the more so in view of the abnormality, and was tempted to offer drug therapy for anxiety and depression. He wondered if he should ask the health visitor to call on Mrs Bellamy at home to see how she was coping with Kerry. The home nurse might be able to offer some help in the care of the eventrated bladder. Mr Bellamy was poorly paid as a semi-skilled worker—perhaps the social worker could ensure that his wife was budgeting sensibly and had enough money to pay the fares to the rather distant special institution where the decisions were to be made about what operations should be performed. Since Mrs Bellamy was anxious to have another baby perhaps genetic counselling should be offered to her and her husband.

The doctor decided for the moment to offer none of these forms of help. He did not feel that he understood enough to enable him to predict how Mrs Bellamy would see any of them. Why had she been so desperate to get pregnant immediately she got married? Why had she married a man 20 years older than herself? Why was she so eager to get pregnant again so quickly? Why was she so neat and efficient in handling Kerry and so drab and untidy herself? What was making her anxious? Was it only the ectopic bladder, about which she appeared to know more than the doctor himself did?

Seeking answers to these questions, the doctor encouraged Mrs Bellamy to talk more about herself. She said that her mother and father had separated when she was 6 years old. She had seen her father only twice after that in the seven years that went by before her mother married again. She had begun her first period on her mother's wedding day. Her mother had never talked to her about menstruation. She had met her future husband when she was 16, just after her mother had given birth to her half-brother. 'I had to have a baby as soon as I got married. I wanted something of my own to love.'

The doctor decided that Mrs Bellamy saw herself as incomplete and unloved, a picture which would have been confirmed by her feeling that she could not even produce a proper baby. She would have to live with the evidence of this for many years. He felt that his objective in treatment should be to encourage her obvious competence in caring for Kerry by allowing his admiration for her abilities to show. He decided not to use any of the other resources which were available to him, nor would he give Mrs Bellamy any drugs for herself. Such actions might all be necessary in due course, but at this first consultation it seemed to him that to take them would only confirm Mrs Bellamy in her illness, which was what her distorted picture of herself amounted to. He would accept, for the moment, Mrs Bellamy's visits with Kerry at their face value and use them as opportunities to carry out his long-term plans.

Illness unorganised

The hoary old joke 'What's the trouble?'—'That's what I've come to find out' has considerable point to it. As first-contact doctor, the general practitioner may have to bring together information from any and every area of a patient's life to define the nature of his problems in such a way that it is possible to discern a helpful response. In this sense, the task is not so much to 'take' a history as to create one.

Even at the more mundane level of describing the progress of obvious organic disease, the 'history' is often modified by the process of talking about it.

> Mr Cramble, aged 79, 'was never ill'. He asked for a visit one evening because he had had nausea and vomiting for six days. The doctor found him mildly dehydrated, rather greyish-yellow in colour, pyrexial and with an equivocal Murphy's sign. He had not had any pain, his urine was normal and his stools had been a normal colour although very loose. He would not go to hospital, but he agreed to a domiciliary consultation the next day. When the surgeon came, Mr Cramble gave him a classical story of gall-stone colic, with pale stools and dark urine—though he had not had any pain since the day before.

The questions that the general practitioner had asked, and the time-interval, had given the patient a chance to sort out a coherent story.

Beyond the difficulties of organising the history lies the possibility of organising the illness itself. 'Psychosomatic' is a loosely used term, best reserved for conditions with visible pathological changes and evidence that emotions play an important part in initiating them. It now seems quite likely that some forms of cancer fall into this category; illness of any sort is commoner after bereavement; and there is room for speculation about the feelings of vague malaise that sometimes precede serious medical conditions. It is therefore conceivable that the way illness is first organised may have a bearing on which pathological processes are set in train; and even that refusing to organise feelings of illness before some transitional stage is reached could be preventive medicine of the highest order.

Such speculation apart, helping people to alter their habits and learn to abandon neurotic ways of thinking and behaving may have the most important effects on their health many years later. The continuing personal care that general practice can provide, undertaken with imagination, makes changing the future in these ways possible. This is what we mean by 'using the doctor-patient relationship'.

Demands upon the doctor

The discipline imposes many demands upon the doctor. He must resist the temptation to be as all-knowing as he is often asked to be; tolerate uncertainty while always seeking to enlarge his knowledge; act consistently within whatever role he sees as therapeutic; and be aware that all his actions affect and are affected by his relationship with his patients.

This book is intended to help those who read it to see more clearly the realities and possibilities that lie within those relationships, and to support those who fear that plunging into the dark waters of their patients' feelings will make them less effective. So often the first attempts are followed by Pandora's cry 'But what can I do now?' We believe that the study of relationships brings not only a measure of understanding, but also a recognition of practical ways in which patients can be helped.

2

The relationship

A relationship may begin before the participants in it meet each other. What one knows about the other before their first meeting affects it and so do the circumstances in which they meet. Prior knowledge and circumstances create expectations.

Expectations and their origin

Mr Abel, an elderly American, had undergone a prostatectomy in New York five weeks before he consulted the English general practitioner to whom he had been recommended. He was in considerable pain from urinary retention, probably due to a urethral stricture from the indwelling catheter used post-operatively, and now exacerbated by a urinary infection. The doctor explained what he thought had happened and said he would arrange an immediate specialist consultation with a view to catheterisation, treatment of any infection confirmed, and later urethral dilatation if it proved necessary. Mr Abel, irritated by the way his trip to England was being spoiled, was quite unable to understand why he had to see another doctor and waste even more time. He had, after all, been recommended by his own doctor to see the English general practitioner if things went wrong after his prostatectomy. Wasn't the English doctor competent, and if he wasn't why should Mr Abel take his advice?

Mr Abel had a clear understanding of the functions of different doctors in his own New York society, and the origin of his expectations is clear. Differences in expectation between people from the same country are harder to predict.

At his first surgery session in a new practice the doctor was consulted by a 20-year-old woman. Mrs Bates was worried about the vaginal bleeding which had begun three weeks after her D & C for an incomplete abortion. It had been her first pregnancy. Although all the indications were that this was a menstrual loss, the doctor thought it essential to perform a vaginal examination and explained his reasons for doing so. After telling Mrs Bates that the os was closed, he encouraged her to talk of her feelings about the miscarriage and to say if she had any fears about future pregnancies. As she reached the door, Mrs Bates turned and asked, 'Whom do I see when I get pregnant again?' 'Whichever partner you wish,' replied the doctor, very aware that he was new to the practice and was acting almost as a locum. 'I won't be able to see you, I suppose. You're a specialist, aren't you?' The doctor called

6

Mrs Bates back to explain this cryptic statement. It turned out that Mrs Bates had never been examined vaginally by a male general practitioner before: she was accustomed to practices in which female doctors did all the gynaecology and obstetrics.

Mrs Bates's expectations were different from those of her new general practitioner and, indeed, each doctor differs in what he expects of himself. If a patient is to gain maximum benefit from a consultation it seems essential for a general practitioner to be able to vary his style of consulting, at least enough to elicit and adapt to the patient's expectations.

Expectations and preferences

Because a patient has expectations about how doctors will behave, it does not mean that he necessarily likes what he expects.

> Miss Cable was a 22-year-old newly-registered patient. In an educated accent she introduced herself, explained that she was trying to complete her Ph.D. thesis, but that she was having trouble sleeping and wanted some more of the sleeping tablets which she had been taking for several months. The doctor replied that he was rather unhappy about prescribing sleeping tablets over long periods of time and needed to know a little bit more before he could give them. Miss Cable appeared astonished and rather angry. She told the doctor that she had originally discussed her problems with her supervisor, who had suggested, to her surprise, that she get some sleeping tablets. She had now become used to them and found herself quite unable to get a good night's sleep without them, though she felt 'pretty dopey' in the mornings. In the end she left, satisfied by an explanation of withdrawal effects, to try out some simple behavioural techniques.

Expectations on both sides

Each of the three stories used so far in this chapter has illustrated that the quality of a doctor-patient relationship is determined by the expectations of the patients. Sometimes it is the doctor's expectations that create a problem.

> Mrs Dale, a 30-year-old speech therapist, had had a series of unfortunate events after the birth of her first child ten months earlier. Her antenatal care and delivery had been arranged privately. She had breast-fed her son and had attributed her continuing amenorrhoea to this until she began to feel nauseated. A pregnancy test by a pharmacist had been positive and she had then obtained a termination through a private non-profit-making organisation. A little later, pains in the iliac fossae were attributed by 'her gynaecologist' to salpingitis and treated as such. Then she had had a laparoscopy at which a chocolate cyst had been found and aspirated. All this had been achieved without consulting her general practitioner and had involved a number of absences from home. Now she brought her 10-month-old James because he was crying at night and wouldn't settle. She wanted to be referred to a paediatrician she had heard about: would the doctor give her a letter as they couldn't afford more private care and the paediatrician would not accept a self-referral.

The doctor was affected by her story but annoyed because Mrs Dale appeared to have complete contempt for his own competence. A woman whom he saw as in dire need of a supportive doctor-patient relationship was behaving in a way so contrary to his expectations that he hardly knew how to begin.

Expectations about outcome

The belief that modern medicine can perform miracles often gives rise to expectations that the doctor sees as unrealistic.

At first sight it may seem that a patient should feel pleased and reassured at being told: 'I'm glad to say that I can find nothing wrong.' Most doctors regard 'reassurance' as a prime part of their function. On further consideration it becomes obvious why 'nothing wrong' is not always the best possible news: it means that the doctor can't 'make' the patient better.

> Mrs Eames, a 38-year-old West Indian, came into the consulting room on a warm spring day wearing a turban-like hat. She said shyly that she was going bald and asked if the doctor would help her. Her records showed that she had been referred the previous year to a dermatologist who had concluded that Mrs Eames had the female equivalent of male baldness, and that nothing at all could be done for her. When she removed her turban, the doctor saw that she had a receding hair-line and central thinning. Her embarrassment was understandable, and she was not better off learning that nothing abnormal was uncovered by the tests which the doctor repeated.

Even learning of the *likelihood* that nothing abnormal will be found is a disappointment, especially in fields where 'miracles' are frequently reported in the newspapers and on television.

> Mr and Mrs Fair, both aged 28, consulted their doctor because conception had not occurred within 14 months of 'stopping all precautions'. They were both intelligent and well-informed about the steps which would be taken to check their fertility. The doctor discussed these with them, but sensed that the pressure of their joint anxiety had a desperate quality. 'In most couples who fail to conceive no abnormality is found,' he began, in an attempt to reassure them. Mrs Fair's face fell. 'Oh dear,' she said, 'I had hoped you *would* find something wrong because then you would have been able to correct it.'

Mrs Fair's logic was impeccable only if anything found to be wrong could be easily corrected. When the doctor said this to her, she replied, 'If doctors can make test-tube babies, they ought to be able to deal with minor problems.' Mrs Fair had been deceived by the image of modern medicine projected by the media, which implies that almost anything can be corrected if only it can be diagnosed.

Expectations and self-respect

People are often justifiably confused about how doctors expect them to behave: 'Do not waste the doctor's time with trivialities,' but 'Do not delay presenting symptoms that may be serious;' and 'It was sensible of you to consult me about this,' but 'Now follow my instructions exactly.' These are but two examples of inconsistent expectations by doctors that can impair the doctor-patient relationship.

Testing expectations

The importance of 'reality-testing' extends far beyond its use by psychiatrists engaged in diagnosing psychosis: we all need to be able to distinguish what is real from what is not real. Even a baby learns that his thumb does not bring him the same reward as a nipple.

Patients often need to test how real their expectations are. 'I know you'll think I'm being silly doctor, but . . .' is a phrase heard in almost every consulting session. The doctor should ask himself three questions: 'Are the reported events real?', 'What beliefs is the patient testing?' and 'What is the patient really frightened about—that his beliefs are true, or that he is losing his ability to distinguish between reality and fantasy?'

Lay beliefs about health

As research into the doctor-patient relationship continues, it becomes clear that most people have well-systematised beliefs about how symptoms are related to each other, against which they test the value of the explanations, advice or treatment given them by doctors.

Mr Greaves, aged 55, a labourer, limped into the consulting room to complain that his left leg was swollen. The doctor found oedema up to the knee, a grossly infected foot and large tender lymph nodes in the left groin, but the right leg was normal. During the examination Mr Greaves said complacently, 'It's all right doctor, I came before the swelling got above the knee. I've been holding the swelling in check by getting up and pissing three times every night.' The doctor felt more than a little confused until Mr Greaves went on to explain that if leg-swelling gets above the knee the fluid enters the veins and begins to drown the heart; passing urine reduces swelling and protects the heart.

Mr Greaves's beliefs bore considerable resemblance to medical views about congestive cardiac failure and its treatment, but he went wrong because the situation in which he applied them was not what he thought it to be.

Mrs Halliwell visited the doctor for the first time in four years, and after a few false starts, closed her eyes and said with a rush 'Doctor, can you tell, I mean do you have any definite kind of feelings or symptoms or anything when you get a brain tumour?' She went on to explain that not only did she look very like her mother—she had also had an uncannily similiar life. Both had had a handicapped child, both had been widowed in their thirties and both had had their gall-bladders removed in their forties. Mrs Halliwell had reached the age of 51, one year younger than her mother had been when she developed a glioblastoma; she was suffering from headaches, insomnia, attacks of dizziness and an inability to concentrate. Sometimes she thought that these symptoms were the product of her fears, but increasingly often it seemed possible that they were early signs of her brain tumour. 'I don't think I'd mind so much if it was the worst—I know what I'd do. What I can't stand is not knowing what's happening to me. It's like my own brain's playing tricks on me and it's driving me out of my mind!'

Expectations and roles

Many of the stories quoted in this chapter could be used to illustrate 'role-theory', a sociologist's perspective which studies the extent to which people's behaviour is determined by the role they are playing at the time. Role-behaviour is most likely to occur between people who do not know each other, and it is no coincidence that, in most of these stories, the doctor and the patient were meeting for the first time. As their relationship becomes more intimate, both doctor and patient find it easier to behave, and allow the other to behave, according to their idiosyncratic attitudes and personalities; but roles do continue to exert an effect. One aspect of role which can never be ignored concerns the authority of the doctor in a professional relationship.

Power, authority, and control

Throughout this book we make the assumption that it is the doctor's professional responsibility to do his best for the patient, and that this 'best' will involve judgements about the patient's perceptions as well as his needs. These judgements must take into account as much information as possible, and this includes information about the nature of the doctor-patient relationship. The role of doctor carries a degree of power, authority and control which puts the patient's independence as an individual at risk whenever the doctor extends his considerations beyond the presenting symptom or the routine response.

Mr Imber, a 25-year-old accountant, complained of rectal soreness. He had discussed with the doctor on an earlier occasion the loneliness of his life since he had moved to the big city, and how this was compounded by being a homosexual. Mr Imber was suffering from urethritis, looked unwell and had some conjunctivitis, as well as pains in the joints. Inspection of the perianal area showed not only the characteristic 'funnelling' of the area but also some blebs. The doctor was concerned to define whether or not his patient had Reiter's syndrome or gonorrhoea. He questioned Mr Imber about his recent sexual activities, only to have him burst into tears about the recent break-up of what had seemed a happy homosexual relationship. 'Can we come back to that on another occasion, Mr Imber?' said the doctor. 'My concern now is to make sure that we find out precisely what is wrong with you, and I'll need the help of a hospital to be certain you get appropriate treatment.'

There can be no doubt that the doctor was controlling the direction of this consultation; that he intended to benefit his patient by doing so does not alter the fact. The right to exert this kind of control may have one of two origins. One can be termed 'authority', something donned with the costume of the role: it relates to the beliefs of a society about someone's right to control the behaviour of others. Certainly the role 'doctor' carries with it this kind of right. Paradoxically, his authority must often be given up if the doctor is to gain what we can call 'power'. Power is something freely accorded by one individual to another and is idiosyncratic to the relationship between them; it stems from a judgement of the person who gives it about the other person's competence and motives. Not only is it given freely, it may be taken away again if the judgement is altered when circumstances change.

Failure of the part of the doctor to distinguish between the two kinds of control can have troublesome consequences.

Mr Jarrett, a 46-year-old divorced plumber, had registered with the practice at the beginning of July, ten weeks before he stormed into the doctor's consulting room. 'Why won't you and your partners give me enough of my tablets?' he asked angrily. The doctor had been presented with a request for a repeat prescription of an analgesic combination, but the medical records had not been received from the FPC. The practice notes showed requests every ten days for prescriptions of what seemed excessive quantities of the tablets. The notes were annotated in red to the effect that Mr Jarret appeared depressed, that investigations were said to reveal no organic cause for the severe occipital headaches which had plagued him for two years, and that he now seemed to be addicted to his analgesic combination. An anti-depressant had been prescribed, together with a calculated quantity of the analgesic. 'I keep having to see different doctors and none of you gives me enough of my tablets. The new tablets don't work at all. I knew they wouldn't!' The doctor apologised for the number of doctors involved, blaming it on doctors' holidays, which was partly true, rather than on Mr Jarrett's demand always to be seen urgently. He went on to make an observation about how angry Mr Jarrett seemed to be, and asked if Mr Jarrett understood the doctors' reluctance to prescribe the quantities of analgesic tablets which he had requested. 'I suppose they don't believe I have the pain. One of your partners accused me of being an addict. I *do* have the pain and it wasn't *my* idea to have the tablets in the first place: the hospital prescribed them when the specialists said they couldn't help me in any other way. I *have* to take twice the quantity because the pain comes back otherwise. The tablets are only pain-killers after all. I'd sooner not have the pain at all.' The doctor explained what a minimum lethal dose was and that for the tablets concerned the therapeutic dose was sufficiently close to make them unsuitable treatment for pain as severe and intractable as Mr Jarrett's appeared to be. 'If I'd understood *that*,' said Mr Jarrett, 'I'd sooner have had the pain than take the risk. I thought your partners were just calling me neurotic and didn't believe that I really had the pain.'

Mr Jarrett was, of course, correct in part. The doctors had been correct in part, too. A good deal of Mr Jarrett's pain seemed relieved when the doctor manipulated his neck. The patient had seen the other doctors' decisions to control his tablets as an exercise of their authority, and his resentment had obscured the way he presented his symptoms. The doctor's explanation seemed to move the relationship from one related only to social role to a more intimate one where some power was given to the doctor because his good intentions had become clear. The change may have been partly responsible for the 'magical' effect of the neck manipulation and the exercises which were suggested to follow it.

Describing the relationship

Describing a relationship as 'good' means almost nothing, except perhaps to indicate that it conforms to the prejudices of the speaker about what such relationships should be like. The attempt by Szasz & Hollender (1956) to use categories based on dominance, co-operation and mutual participation takes things a little further but still over-simplifies them too much to be useful.

In real life the possibilities are infinite and their number cannot be reduced. To put into words what happens to every conflict, confrontation, collusion, coming together or new venture, whether hidden or overt, in a consultation would require qualities of sensitivity and expression that very few people possess. Nevertheless, it is clear from experience that many medical students and doctors do need some kind of guide, if only to stimulate their imaginations.

We have chosen to use 'harmony' as our central concept, though there are many alternatives—intimacy, honesty or warmth, for instance. We then have to add the dimension of 'appropriateness', since two people may be in perfect harmony while playing the wrong tune.

Harmony

When there is harmony, doctor and patient have the same assumptions about how *each* should behave; in addition, the patient is happy about the doctor's emotional response to his story. At this level the nature of these behaviours is irrelevant, though for other purposes they may need to be described.

Few doctors are so rigid that they do not vary their behaviour according to the patient's age, sex, social class and other characteristics; in conjunction with the tolerance that most patients display, this probably provides enough flexibility to make doctors' behaviour acceptable more often than not. There may well be less agreement about acceptable behaviour in patients, though this can only be a matter for speculation.

If the response that the doctor shows matches that which the patient hoped to evoke, then what the doctor communicates in return is likely to be agreeable to the patient.

Apparent harmony
There are times when neither the doctor not the patient wants the lack of harmony between them to become apparent. A patient may find the doctor patronising, peremptory or over-sympathetic, for instance, but be prepared to swallow his feelings because he believes that the doctor is technically competent and well-intentioned, or because no other doctor is available. A doctor may conceal irritation or distaste because he believes that he should always do so, because he wants to project a particular image, or because he does not want to provoke aggression, withdrawal or tears. 'Assumed' harmony can occur when one party is not listening to what the other is saying.

Disharmony
Doctor and patient may disagree about many things—roles, statuses, what they should be talking about, or how seriously or intimately they should talk, for example. This is bound to be uncomfortable, and it may result in a breakdown of communications, but it need not do so. Overt disagreement can be acknowledged and often resolved, though if this is not done thoroughly the outcome is likely to be only an apparent harmony.

Apparent disharmony
Some marriages seem to to an outsider to flourish on, or despite, an extraordinary level of conflict, and the equivalent situation is sometimes found in doctor-patient relationships. Presumably there is an underlying harmony which is heard only by the couple.

Neutrality
Often it would be truer to say that doctor and patient have no special feelings about each other than that their views are in harmony. This state of affairs could be called neutrality, and is most likely

to be found when their business together has been brief, superficial and largely concerned with matters not in dispute. This need not be the case, for it is quite conceivable that a patient could tell a story of considerable emotional intensity without having significant feelings about the doctor—as particularly sympathetic, suspicious or uninterested, for example. Apparent neutrality may exist too, but distinguishing it from apparent harmony would be difficult.

Appropriateness
A relationship is appropriate when it helps the patient get what he needs (as distinct from wants). It is inappropriate if it impedes this essential result of a consultation.

Once it is accepted that a doctor-patient relationship can affect clinical outcome, it is clear that the doctor has a responsibility to exert some conscious control over its nature. A teacher who sets out to influence the way his pupil thinks has a similar responsibility, because he is also trying to bring a permanent change, and parents have a much greater responsibility of the same kind to their children. Deliberate manipulation is distasteful in social relationships, where there is no assumption of responsibility, but it is permissible in a professional relationship.

It follows that the doctor should not allow his relationship with a patient to become too defined until he has a good understanding of what the patient needs (as distinct from wants) from it—any more than he would offer his collection of drug samples to a patient to choose from before he has made a diagnosis. The time it takes to achieve this understanding varies.

Mrs Drabble (Chapter 4) aroused the sympathy of her doctor and had a harmonious relationship with him in which they agreed that she was an unfortunate victim of circumstances who needed a constant supply of transquillisers. She then met another doctor who did not share her feelings and was not frightened of disharmony; he gave her a chance to mature by challenging her painfully, appropriately and immediately.

The doctor saw quickly that Mr Appleyard (Chapter 10) needed someone who carried great power and self-confidence to help him change his way of life, and behaved accordingly.

Assessment of a patient's needs cannot always be made so early on a relationship. Sometimes the doctor may, while keeping his options open, play a hunch. When Mrs Burns (Chapter 12) asked for a repeat prescription of her sleeping tablets, the doctor sensed that she wanted him to resist despite her protestations to the contrary. It turned out that her chief need was for support while the process of 'health breaking through' was taking place, so that he was given a clue to the kind of relationship that he needed to foster, through periods of great difficulty, from the first consultation.

In the story of Mrs Childs, described at length in Chapter 7, it was all that the doctor could do to hang on for two years without closing any doors, guided only by the belief that she needed to learn how to manage her relationships better. By remaining interested, but keeping a low profile, he eventually enabled her to trust him with secrets that were very important to her, and the shape of their future relationship began to form. Even then, it was far from clear to him how he should try to use the power Mrs Childs had given him in directing their relationship for her future benefit.

In modern general practice patients are not always able to see the same doctor for every consultation, and the records should convey something of the patient's beliefs, assumptions and expectations if it is to be a useful guide to other people who may be called upon to give professional help. They will also need some indication of how the doctor sees the doctor-patient relationship and what he hopes to achieve through it—comments that the doctor can use himself when he is trying to review where he has got to. A method and a language for recording information like this is as much of a practical necessity as a proper system for displaying data of a more traditional medical kind. The concepts of harmony and appropriateness could form a useful starting place.

Reference

Szasz T, Hollender M 1956 A contribution to the philosophy of medicine: basic models of the doctor-patient relationship. Archives of Internal Medicine 97: 585

3

Assumptions

In the previous chapter a few consultations were presented in which differing beliefs by doctor and patient about the relative roles of general practitioner and specialist caused difficulties; more subtle differences can have even greater effects. Any relationship can be complicated by mismatching assumptions that remain unspoken; the transactions in a consultation, laden as they often are with fear, anger, desperation or guilt, have special risks attached to them.

Everyone must make assumptions, if only to avoid being overwhelmed by a welter of experiences which he can never fully explore; the sum of his assumptions has been called his 'assumptive world'. Many problems are presented to a general practitioner which arise because a patient's assumptive world differs from that of the people round him; the general practitioner must ensure, as far as he can, that further problems are not created by the effects of his own assumptions. The responsibility is especially pressing since it is in general practice that the nature of patients' problems is first defined in medical terms.

The closer we are to any patient in nationality, colour, age, sex, education and social background, the more our assumptive world is likely to resemble his, but many assumptions are based on personal factors like unconscious needs and unique experiences which the patient may repress. We need to recognise our own assumptions so that we may avoid acting carelessly, and as many as we can of our patients' assumptions to avoid acting inappropriately.

Why patients consult

In theory, professional and public assumptions about the functions of the general practitioner in our system match pretty well. He is there to decide whether or not a patient's symptoms have a medical cause, and to diagnose and deal with them if they do; to advise people about matters of health and illness; to support patients whose conditions are incurable; to offer accepted preventive measures; and, when necessary, to provide access to the many services and benefits that require his signature. There would also be pretty general agreement that patients should avail themselves of these functions in a sensible and responsible way.

Such broad theoretical agreement does not preclude differences of opinion and assumption at a practical level, and these will be considered below, but there are some areas in which even theoretical agreement is not complete. Psychosocial problems are a good example: to many doctors and many members of the public they are the province of every reasonable and compassionate general practitioner, while others, from both camps, believe either that they waste a doctor's time and training or that he should not deal with them because doing so adds to the medicalisation of everyday life. Broad social trends are reducing the discrepancy, and so too is scientific progress. Nothing is more likely to medicalise a condition than a new drug which claims to cure or alleviate it.

Patients do not go to their doctors only for the socially-defined reasons mentioned above. Many of the most baffling consultations which put such a strain on the doctor-patient relationship are better understood in other terms: the advantage they offer a patient in his relationship with others, or the chance they give him to play Games (see Chapter 9); sometimes they can be construed best as an habitual response to anxiety of any kind.

We believe that particular attention must be paid to the assumptions which the doctor and the patient make about each other, about what is normal, about what the 'real' problem is and about what should happen.

Assumptions about each other

R. D. Laing's *Knots* succinctly classifies the nature and consequences of the false assumptions that people make about each other. His three levels can be summarised as:

The view that each has of the other
The view that each feels the other has of him
What the first feels that the second believes is the first's view of him (and vice versa)

In more concrete terms, and using feelings about 'listening' as an example, the three levels would be:

'He's not listening to me'
'He thinks I'm not listening to him'
'He thinks I don't believe he's listening to me'

Neither doctor nor patient is likely to be happy if he thinks that the other is not listening to him. Examples of first level effects can be found in case-histories quoted elsewhere in this book: Mrs Entwistle's gall-stone colic was missed for a long time because she made the doctor feel too hopeless to hear what she was saying (Chapter 5); while the mutual liking and respect for one another of Mr Coghill and his doctor (Chapter 6) produced a situation in which Mr Coghill could get the sympathetic support he needed.

The second level is well illustrated by contrasting the thoughts and feelings of the doctor with those of the patient about the patient's symptoms. The patient sees them in a personal context and often has no idea of their clinical significance; the doctor is naturally more detached—he sees many people with similar complaints and has a professional knowledge of what they are likely to mean. Each may sense that there is some conflict between their respective points of view, and feel irritated, frustrated and misunderstood as a result.

The third level accounts for many instances of breakdown in communication. A patient who displays some irritation when the doctor repeats a piece of advice several times can irritate the doctor who does not believe that the patient has fully understood its importance, yet feels blocked by the patient's reaction from giving it again. In the opposite direction, the doctor may be impatient at repetition by a patient while the patient is still not convinced that the doctor really understands what he is trying to say, and both get bad feelings. The block may need to be acknowledged and discussed.

What is normal

Wendy Acheson, aged 22, came into the consulting room, and before she had even reached the chair, said to the doctor 'The bastard! He's done it again!'

It appeared that her husband had just told her that he had been found to have gonorrhoea, and wanted her to get some treatment. It was the third time that this happened, and on each occasion the infection had followed one of his business trips to Birmingham.

'What are you going to do?' asked the doctor. 'I suppose I'd better have some more Septrin.' Thinking of the problems that even one such announcement might have caused in some marriages, the doctor was a little surprised at her reaction.

Wendy Acheson seemed to expect men to behave like this. Her expectations may have been determined by the 'sub-culture' of her environment, just as the behaviour of the young man in the next story may have been learned in his family; in both cases it is arguable that basic personality factors were more important.

Michael Burford, aged 24, consulted the doctor and said very calmly 'You'll think I'm crazy, doctor, but could you let me have some tranquillisers?' He was managing a shop where the owner was present all the time; when there was any difference of opinion, for example over an invoicing or delivery mistake, the boss would apparently become very excited and start shouting. 'He's driving me mad, doctor.' Mr Burford had found another job and was going to give in his notice. 'Look, doctor, I'm terrified of what's going to happen when I tell him. He'll go mad and he'll make life unbearable.' Not working out his notice would spoil his future prospects.

The doctor commented that the patient seemed to believe that anger should be completely controlled, while the boss preferred to let it out. He noticed that the patient had assumed he would be thought mad asking for transquillisers and was probably wondering if the doctor would accept the reason he had given. In the end they decided that the best solution would be a doctor's note stating that the patient was leaving his employment on medical advice.

The boss telephoned the doctor the next day. When the doctor explained that he could not discuss the matter, he said 'I suppose it's because I fly off the handle so easily. If I don't, I get so tense I can't work at all.'

Their conflicting assumptions about the expression of anger made a continuing relationship between the young man and his boss impossible. In the next case the conflict was between doctor and patient.

Mrs Charnley, aged 35, had a fourth child seven years after her third. When the baby was 11 months old the mother complained at the well-baby clinic that he still dirtied his nappies. When the doctor said 'Of course he does,' Mrs Charnley disagreed: 'My others were clean at that age.' The doctor expressed his doubts, adding that in his experience babies might be clean in the sense that their motions could be collected in a pot after a feed, but that they could not deliberately wait for the pot to be presented. In any case, most babies would lose this regularity before acquiring bowel control and so would begin to have dirty nappies again. Mrs Charnley seemed to accept this explanation.

A week later his partner said jokingly to him 'I hear you had an awful job getting your children clean when they were babies,' and went on to tell him that Mrs Charnley had just consulted him about the same problem. She had commented that his partner accepted dirty nappies because he had had trouble with his own children, but she knew that there was something wrong with her baby, whatever the doctor might think was normal.

The mother's assumptions in this case were not easy to reconcile with reality. Possibly she was angry that the first doctor had implied that she was either stupid or crazy; in any case he had made it impossible for her to learn from him.

The next story illustrates a culture-bound assumption which the doctor recognised from his experience of many patients from related cultures.

Mr Duleep, a 32-year-old Sikh, complained of vague pains in his neck and shoulders. The doctor said 'You look worried.' Taking a deep breath, the patient replied 'I am having nocturnal discharge—it is weakening, isn't it?' Knowing that Hindus believe the conserving of semen to be necessary for good health, the doctor asked if it were the same for Sikhs. The patient said it was for him. The doctor asked about contact with women, and the patient told him that his wife was still in India. He had been to prostitutes when he had first come to England, but not in the last few years. The doctor assured him that his discharges would do him no harm, and that they would probably continue as long as he was not having intercourse. Since he might catch a venereal disease from a prostitute it might be better to accept them until his wife could join him. 'It's really a sign of how much of a man you are.'

The dangers we have mentioned so far are those of not picking up and discussing differing assumptions, and those of being irritated by an assumption thought to be false. There is a further danger: that the doctor will adopt the patient's assumption when it should be challenged. An illustrative case-history is that of Mrs Edwards in Chapter 6.

One special example of differing assumptions about what is normal is described in Chapter 12 as the syndrome of 'health breaking through', in which the symptoms that are causing the patient to assume that he is ill are interpreted by the doctor as a sign of returning normality. Here, and in other cases where an attempt is being made to persuade someone to relinquish an assumption, a combination of reason, persuasiveness and flexibility is required. These are the elements of a process of negotiation, undertaken so that doctor and patient may start from shared premises about the nature of what is happening. In the case of Mrs Charnley no such negotiations took place.

What is the 'real' problem

The idea that the presenting problem may not be the most important problem is familiar to everyone, but so too is the story of the woman who complains 'If you go in there with just a cold, he starts asking you all about your sex life.' The 'real' problem has not only to be defined accurately, it also has to be agreed by the patient. Conflicting assumptions produce stalemate.

Mrs Easton brought her 6-year-old son, John, to the surgery and, with tight lips, said 'Doctor, I'd like you to examine his hair,' The doctor did so and responded 'Yes, he's got some nits there.' He then explained how to get rid of them.

Guessing from her expression that she felt she was being accused of negligence or of having a dirty home, he casually mentioned how one of his own children had been much more resistant to treatment than the others when they had had the same thing. Her response showed that his assumption had been correct and at the end of the consultation she suggested spontaneously that she ought to inform John's school.

The doctor had relied on her making the apparently more powerful assumption that negligence and dirt were inconceivable in a medical household! No such stratagem was available in the next case-history.

> Mrs French, aged 39, came to the surgery complaining of pains in the chest, a thumping heart and dizziness. She asked to be examined and started taking her blouse off while still speaking. The doctor put some more questions to her as she got on to the couch, and she watched his face closely as he put his stethoscope on her chest. She did not seem relieved when he said 'Well, your heart's fine, if that's what's worrying you.' and she was obviously reluctant to get up.
> The doctor asked he if she was under any kind of stress. 'If you think it's just my nerves, I'm not imagining it, doctor!' She denied having any worries and pushed him into arranging an ECG and chest X-ray that he considered diagnostically unnecessary. Even when these showed no abnormality she was unsatisfied. 'Don't you think I ought to see a heart specialist if you don't know what's the matter with me?'

There was no common ground between them about the cause of her symptoms, and the doctor could think of no better plan than to include in his referral letter a request to the cardiologist to reassure her as strongly as possible that her heart was normal.

The idea of negotiating an agreement with the patient was mentioned earlier in connection with assumptions about what is normal, and is even more relevant here. Nothing can be effectively treated unless there is agreement about what should be treated.

The good negotiator needs a clear idea of what he can realistically hope to achieve and the flexibility to subordinate his immediate wishes to objectives of a longer term. He has to take into account how both sides see the situation and what minimum needs each has to satisfy if the relationship is to continue.

The negotiating process in general practice is not usually very explicit; more often it is a matter of doctor and patient finding out what the other will tolerate until a working understanding is reached.

> Jenny Garner, a new patient aged 30, asked for a large supply of Doriden, saying she needed to take four tablets every night. It emerged that she had left her husband and baby daughter eight years earlier and come to London. There she had mixed with hard-drug users, become dependent on barbiturates and amphetamine, and started taking heroin. A stormy period had followed in which she was admitted to hospital several times, once at least because of a serious suicide attempt. After that she had settled in a regular job and learned to manage on 'only' four Doriden tablets a night—an achievement of which she was proud. She was quite unable to form lasting relationships: as soon as there was any danger of one developing she would walk out, or behave so badly that the other person did so instead.
> The doctor was unhappy about the prescription she wanted, but thought that

given a little time he might be able to wean off her hypnotics. He said he would prescribe for her on condition that she agreed to reduce the nightly dose by half a tablet each month. It proved quite easy to get her down to two tablets, but more difficult to reach one and a half; nearly a year later further reduction has never been maintained for more than a month.

The agreement that they now have contains the following elements: the doctor will go on pushing her to cut down; she will not protest as long as no crisis is taking place in her life; there has to be a really good story to warrant an increase from one to one and a half tablets; and no reason for going higher than this will be accepted at all.

She uses the doctor as someone she can talk to about the many crises that come upon her—not to ask for advice but because it helps her formulate what to do about them. When she goes on holiday she always sends him a postcard. The doctor thinks that this relationship is valuable enough to her to make some further reduction of the tablets possible, but since she is never ill it bears little resemblance to the traditional role-relationship of doctor and patient. Final weaning may be difficult if the 'need' for a prescription becomes the only way she can justify coming to see him; but when this happens he hopes that he will be able to substitute a drug of less potential danger.

Sometimes negotiations are conducted entirely in the head of one of the parties, as the following case-histories suggest.

Mrs Hillman, an active and independent woman of 74, lived alone and had not seen a doctor for four years. She visited the surgery complaining of a cough which she had had for a week. The doctor thought she had a minor viral infection, but noted that she seemed more tired than he remembered. He asked about her life in general and after telling him about her many problems she seemed to brighten up and look more hopeful.

He sensed that she was not going to admit that the 'real' problem was loneliness, so that he could not offer a 'contract' that allowed her to come and talk to him when she felt particularly lonely. Instead he decided to accept her presenting complaint as the 'real' one, and pretend that the more important matters had been brought up incidentally in the course of a social chat. He prescribed a cough medicine not for its dubious pharmacological effects, but to make it easier for her to come back when she wanted to.

It may, on the other hand, be the patient who entertains the silent dialogue.

Mrs Illingworth, aged 54, had not consulted for some years, and was meeting the doctor for the first time. She complained of nocturnal cramps in her calves. Increasing in frequency and severity, they now woke her regularly at about 3.30am, and she could not get back to sleep. It crossed the doctor's mind that this early morning wakening might indicate depression, even though she did not look especially depressed. After considering the cramps he'turned to her emotional state and found definite evidence that confirmed his suspicion. The consultation ended with a prescription for antidepressants and an arrangement to see her frequently in the next few weeks.

A month or so later, Mrs Illingworth told the doctor that she had planned in some detail how she would kill herself after getting home from her first visit to the surgery; she would have implemented the plans if the consultation had not gone the way it did and given her some hope.

Though she had denied suicidal intent in the consultation some negotiated agreement must have been reached with the doctor in her head. Nearly ten years later the doctor still feels acutely uncomfortable about the part played by luck in leading him to the right diagnosis.

Success in negotiating is often a matter of timing. The first concession may need to come from the doctor and involve some departure from his usual way of working.

A general practitioner was asked by one of his partners to see a 67-year-old man called Mr Jamieson who was pretty depressed, but who had refused to accept this to the point where an impasse had been reached.

Mr Jamieson made the necessary appointment and came the next day. He said that his own doctor was very kind but refused to believe that he needed treatment for his bronchitis. The notes confirmed that Mr Jamieson was a chronic bronchitic and the patient said that he knew from past experience that a course of an antibiotic would help him. The doctor reckoned that the circumstances gave him a free hand so he wrote a prescription for ampicillin without further discussion or examination and asked the patient to come back in a week.

Mr Jamieson felt and looked better when he returned. As the doctor was applying his stethoscope he heard the patient mutter 'I didn't think it would come to this.' When they returned to their seats the doctor asked what these words meant. Mr Jamieson told him how proud he had always been of his physical fitness which had saved his life twice during the war; it was hard enough for him to accept his present physical condition which made him feel useless, but when his doctor had implied that he was cracking up mentally as well, this was more than he could bear.

The doctor discovered that he was not in fact useless, since he was looking after his crippled wife very diligently. Mr Jamieson then confirmed how depressed he felt and said that this was making it harder to cope at home. He would be happy to have any treatment that would 'get him going again properly'.

There are many reasons why people may present something other than the 'real' problem. Sometimes they do not know that the latter has any connection with the symptoms they are suffering; sometimes they do not want any help with it apart from symptomatic relief and try to avoid talking about it; and sometimes they need to 'test' the doctor first with something else before deciding to trust him with more important matters.

When the presenting problem seems to be no more than an entry-ticket to the consulting room and is unlikely to be important in its own right, it can often be discarded fairly quickly; on other occasions it may be put to one side, by agreement, until after the more pressing problem has been dealt with. The clue that there is some more pressing problem may come in many different forms: unusual behaviour, like the presentation of a cold by a patient who has not been seen for years; non-verbal cues from the patient's expression, gestures, posture and dress, reflecting an emotional state which he does not mention; and an opening of the consultation by the patient with an apparently general question rather than a statement about his symptoms.

> Mrs King, aged 48, had been on the doctor's list for six months before she
> first consulted him. 'My periods have been irregular, doctor. Could it be the
> change?' The doctor thought it would be sensible, before going into
> gynaecological details, to see what she felt and thought about the menopause,
> and he asked her what it meant to her.
> He soon found out that, whatever her gynaecological condition, a very
> pressing problem lay elsewhere. At the age of 50 her mother had 'gone mad',
> and Mrs King had always been told how like her mother she was. She was
> very frightened that she would soon go mad too; the resulting anxiety was
> giving her symptoms which served to confirm her fears, and she had bottled
> everything up until the doctor's question released it.

Any discussion on negotiation has to consider the times when either arbitration or sanctions may be called for.

Arbitration brings in a third party who should be neutral and respected by both sides, but out-patient appointments made to resolve intractable disagreements between doctor and patient are not always successful. The general practitioner often attempts to bias the specialist's approach, as in the case of Mrs French; the patient is quite likely to believe that doctors tend to stick together and may change his story to create a stronger impression. Non-acceptance of the arbitration by the patient is common—few general practitioners will be surprised to learn that Mrs French was not convinced that her heart was normal, or that she immediately asked to see another specialist. Non-acceptance by the doctor is likely to show itself more subtly.

Both doctor and patient have sanctions available to back up their negotiating. Patients may get 'worse' symptoms, which threaten the doctor's professional self-confidence, or present them more frequently, at more awkward times and in more awkward ways, which threatens the doctor-patient relationship. The doctor's sanctions include not listening, hinting at dire medical consequences, or, even more punitively, offering referral but using a consultant who has a reputation for being rude and authoritarian. The final sanction, of terminating the relationship, is open to both sides, but is used less frequently than one would dare to expect.

In summary, reaching agreement about what is to be treated can be a delicate process the outcome of which depends on the beliefs and feelings of both doctor and patient, and also upon their relationship with each other. The required negotiations may be, at one extreme, completely explicit and, at the other, conducted entirely in the head of one of them. While the presenting problem very often is the 'real' problem, assuming it to be so is sometimes dangerous and always naive. When there is disagreement about which is the 'real' problem it is usually sensible to agree that more than one problem will have to be explored.

One other trap for the unwary exists on those occasions when the doctor is at a loss to account for the symptoms presented. Searching for a psychological explanation has been so emphasised in recent years that, when he discovers an emotional problem, the doctor may be tempted to assume that he has found the cause of the symptoms. This is illogical unless he can establish a clear link between them and the emotional problem; it ignores our still vast ignorance about the physical workings of the body. An admission of ignorance is usually the best policy.

What should happen

A variety of other unwarranted assumptions can bedevil what happens during and after the consultation and affect the doctor-patient relationship.

There are times when a patient's way of understanding things is so conditioned by his previous experience that the doctor's behaviour baffles him. The three case-histories which follow show this happening in different areas.

Mr Logan, a hard-working but rather dull labourer of 38, consulted the doctor about his backache. The doctor had recently learned some of the skills of manipulation and promptly used them. There were some satisfying clicks, and the patient's pain and limitation of movement disappeared.

The doctor sat down to write his notes, expecting some expression of pleasure from the patient; instead he heard, 'Now that's very odd. I can put my clothes on without it hurting me,' followed by a long and awkward silence. Suddenly he realised what was going on in Mr Logan's mind. The man was dressed in his best clothes and knew what happened when you went to the doctor with a genuine backache: you were given painkillers, a certificate to stay off work, and orders to rest completely. The idea of walking out of the room cured was not one to which he could readily adapt.

Mrs Martin, aged 28, presented with symptoms of anxiety. It soon became clear that she had marital problems, and she asked the doctor if he thought she should leave her husband. Since at least part of the trouble seemed to stem from her being too submissive at home, the doctor thought that she should begin to think in terms of making decisions for herself; besides, he felt unqualified to offer that kind of advice. He therefore tried a counselling approach to get her to think more clearly about her situation and the possible ways in which she might do something about it. At the end of the consultation she asked him 'But what do you think I ought to do?' revealing her frustration at getting only questions from him rather than answers and inducing a similar feeling in him.

Mr Nugent, aged 58, came to the surgery to be signed off as fit for work after an attack of influenza. He said he still felt a little run down and would like a 'good old fashioned tonic.' The doctor, judging him to be of reasonable intelligence and ripe for some health education, explained that there was no such thing as a tonic and that he would recover completely without medication in a short time.

Mr Nugent did not take this information well and insisted that a tonic was what he needed; the doctor felt he had burned his boats and could not prescribe something he had already described as useless. The patient went out in a huff and never consulted that doctor again.

At other times it is the doctor who is surprised because he has expectations which derive from his training. For example, doctors differentiate clearly between activities which are designed to produce a diagnosis—history-taking, examination and investigations—and activities which are intended as treatment. Patients do not necessarily make the assumption that these activities are separate. The beneficial effects of a physical examination, a blood test or an X-ray are widely recognised but taking a history can also be therapeutic.

A new trainee told his trainer that he had had a 'very odd consultation indeed' that morning. The patient was a 20-year-old girl called Cheryl Ogden who had complained of feeling tired for the last few weeks. When he had run through his list of systematic questions he had found nothing specific to take as a starting point and the examination had been equally unhelpful. He had told her that he would have to arrange a number of tests to elucidate the problem.

She had agreed to have them and then started to talk about her rather isolated existence as a provincial student in London. The trainee had found her attractive and knew that he had no other patients waiting to see him. He therefore resolved to explore the psychological and social aspects of her life in case the cause of her tiredness lay therein.

About three quarters of an hour had passed with amazing speed when she had said reluctantly that she had to go. He was still no nearer an answer and was relieved that he had at least arranged some investigations. He wanted his trainer to go over the differential diagnosis with him because he felt uneasy, and admitted to feeling a little guilty that the consultation had been enjoyable rather than clinically incisive.

It is not only by providing congenial company that the diagnostic part of the interview can be therapeutic. Patients may value a thorough consideration of their problem, or be reassured when the doctor is not alarmed by what they have told him. The doctor's skill in asking questions that have made them think more clearly, with occasional summaries of what he has understood for them to confirm or correct, can lead them to a new perspective which is helpful. The doctor may think he was engaged only in defining the problem but the patient is way ahead of him in beginning to use the ideas that have occurred to him.

Occasionally patients make assumptions about the purpose of consultations which are hard to justify logically but which the doctor does not necessarily feel to be unreasonable.

Mrs Phillips, a practical and sensible woman of 32, asked the doctor to visit one of her three young children. He had recently seen the eldest with chicken pox. When he arrived he was told 'John has chicken pox now. He's quite well, and I'm using the lotion you gave Peter but I thought you'd want to see him.

However the doctor reacts to this, the consultation certainly cannot be justified on the basis of a need for diagnosis and advice. Finally, doctors make assumptions about 'patient compliance', a term with more than a hint of arrogance in it. Several surveys have shown that doctors assume too frequently that their patients want prescriptions and it is common knowledge that many drugs are either not dispensed or not taken as ordered. It may be unrealistic to regard compliance as a rational behaviour unless either a good reason for it has been negotiated in the consultation or it leads to obvious and immediate relief of the symptoms. Possibly it is only the more obsessional or anxious patient who is disposed to comply and it is evidence of compliance that should give the doctor cause for concern.

4

Understanding and insight

Consultations, no matter what they are about, consist of an exchange of information and assumptions between doctor and patient from which the patient should gain insight into what is the matter with him. This exchange may occupy more than one interview and is never really completed, even in general practice.

Communication has three kinds of intention: *informative* (to convey information), *promotive* (to bring about certain actions) and *evocative* (to arouse certain feelings). It is made non-verbally and para-verbally as well as in words. No nuance of tone, hesitation, posture, movement, expression or appearance can be assumed to be accidental, though it may be unintentional.

When the consultation begins, the doctor can assume only that the patient wants to communicate something; he has all these aspects of the communication to consider before he can apply his professional knowledge. Patients are influenced at least as much by the doctor's non-verbal and para-verbal communications as by what he says, and this affects both what they say and how they say it. To minimise this distorting effect the doctor should not try too hard to limit the range of information that the patient offers him.

Mrs Arden was 34. The doctor had delivered her two children at home and had advised her in the well-baby clinic. He had always felt that she was intelligent and enjoyed chatting with her. When her second baby was 5 months old, Mrs Arden telephoned the doctor to say that her period had lasted for 16 days and had now turned into an unpleasant brown discharge. The doctor suggested that she come to be examined.

She arrived that evening to say, 'It's all right doctor, I've found out the trouble, I had left a Tampax inside me.' She seemed rather upset and went on, 'Isn't it stupid? I've been using them for years and I've never had it happen before.' The doctor said, 'I'm a little surprised; I would have thought there would have been a gap between the stopping of bleeding from a period and the beginning of loss because of a tampon.' 'Oh, there was, doctor! A few days.' The doctor remarked that he was surprised she had not found it when she inserted her cap, knowing that this was the method of birth control she used. 'Oh, we don't have intercourse that often,' said Mrs Arden and got up to go.

She returned three days later looking very distressed. 'I think you doctors have the wrong idea about some things. You implied that most people would have had intercourse after a period finished!' This was exactly what the doctor had implied. 'You're not right, you know! We talked about this where I used to work and a lot of people hardly ever have intercourse. Your idea of what is normal is wrong.' The doctor was a little taken aback. 'It seems to me that you are challenging me to say whether what you and your husband do is normal or abnormal. I don't consider myself the right person to judge that. It may be average in some circles to have intercourse infrequently, but I don't think that you can apply the word normal. It is normal if both you and your husband are satisfied.'

Mrs Arden burst into tears and a completely new set of information was provided.

Uncovering suppressed information

Even when there is an atmosphere that permits the patient to express himself freely, he may suppress information in order to promote certain actions by the doctor. This can confuse the doctor.

> Mrs Blaise, aged 28, came complaining of nausea and vomiting. She did not look well. Could the doctor stop the vomiting, which had happened twice a day for the last three days, as she had to go to her friend's wedding the next day?
>
> No, she had no diarrhoea and her appetite was normal.
>
> Yes, she had abdominal pain, low down.
>
> No, vomiting did not relieve it nor did any particular food upset her.
>
> No, she had never been like this before and no, she had no other symptoms. She just didn't want to be sick at the wedding or the reception.
>
> Well, yes, she was passing water more frequently than usual and she did have some burning discomfort at the end of micturition.
>
> She had severe pyelocystitis, with a temperature of 101°F (38.3°C) and treatment involved her resting and not going to the wedding.

If Mrs Blaise had not looked ill and evoked concern in the doctor she might well have received an anti-emetic rather than treatment for her pyelitis. The doctor stored away the fact that what Mrs Blaise chose to suppress also said something about her sense of social obligation.

It is relatively easy to understand and identify with Mrs Blaise's wish to attend her friend's wedding. Sometimes uncovering suppressed material reveals that the patient is behaving neurotically.

> Mrs Corless was 45, a very sensible woman who managed her family and home easily and well. She came with minimal symptoms of a cold, which was highly unusual behaviour for her. The doctor gave her a prescription but she showed a slight reluctance to leave. When encouraged, Mrs Corless asked if there was anything wrong in having a slight vaginal discharge. The doctor examined her but found no abnormality and indeed no real discharge. With more encouragement, she explained that her mother had died of carcinoma of the cervix at 45 and that she found herself worrying about her own symptoms although she knew that this was silly.

Mrs Corless's behaviour was 'neurotic' in that it was inappropriate to the situation. She was almost more frightened of being thought silly than she was of having carcinoma of the cervix. Luckily there were clues that led the doctor in the right direction so that he was able to give her the reassurance she needed.

The patient's perception of the doctor's assumptions and expectations

Mrs Arden had correctly identified her doctor's assumption that she would have intercourse not many days after the completion of menstruation and felt free to express her anger about this. Some patients (see Chapter 5) will act out their anger at a doctor's unspoken assumptions—which they may, in any case, be misinterpreting.

> Mrs Daiches, a midwife, was 37 weeks pregnant and normally saw the doctor's partner. She called the doctor at 2 am, complaining of pains in the thighs, nausea, palpitations and headaches, and feeling very ill. The doctor received a black look as he entered the bedroom. 'Oh! I thought your partner would come.' 'Did you want to see him?' 'Yes, I wanted to tell him that not all people who have illegitimate babies are to blame. As you're here you had better find out what is wrong with me.'
> The doctor began to examine her and said, 'What on earth did my partner say to upset you so much?' 'Oh, we were talking about all these young girls having illegitimate babies, and he said that most of them knew what they were doing.'
> There followed a full story about her own experience of having an illegitimate baby when she was 17 years old. The baby had died and her father had made her pay him back for the funeral when she was well enough to work again. Now she was having what the partner thought would be her third child at home, but it was really her fourth. She had not wanted it to begin with, but they were Roman Catholic; she knew that risks increased with parity and was afraid something awful would happen.
> The doctor asked her if she felt better now that she had said all this. 'Yes,' she replied, 'but it was really your partner I wanted to tell.' 'Well,' said the doctor, 'either I can tell him for you or you can tell him yourself.' 'I'll go and tell him myself, but it isn't really fair that you've had to get out of bed in the middle of the night because of something your partner said!'

In ordinary conversation many things are left unsaid because they are embarrassing, and this can occur in medical consultations too. It is not surprising that Mrs Arden had not mentioned her sexual problems before, but rather more unexpected that Mrs Daiches should lie about her parity when, as a midwife, she knew its significance, and when her husband was aware of the truth.

Uncovering repressed information

Many doctors view their first clinical task as distinguishing between neurotic and 'real' complaints and feel that neurotic behaviour gets in the way of their attempts to communicate with the patient. When repressed information is uncovered it can be seen that neurotic behaviour is itself a form of communication which becomes understandable when the assumptions on which it is based are made explicit.

> Mary Ellard was 6 years old. Her mother said that Mary had often had abdominal pain which stopped her from going to school. Mary looked very happy but Mrs Ellard looked very worried. 'It's not because she's frightened of school, doctor. She loves it. If I keep her at home she always tells me how much she wants to go, and she does very well there.'
>
> Mary had no physical cause for her pain that the doctor could find. It transpired that Mary worried about her mother when she was in school (a not uncommon phenomenon, analagous to the compulsion of new parents to get up in the night to see if the baby is still breathing). Mary was not frightened of school, but that her mother would come to some harm while she was away. Her method of communicating this was her abdominal pain. The communication was aimed at her mother. It evoked her mother's anxiety and promoted being kept at home. When the doctor told Mrs Ellard his opinion she immediately remembered feeling the same way when she started school although previously she had no memory of it.

Interpretation and insight

Insight is a psychoanalytic concept meaning 'conscious awareness of one's own problem' and it has both emotional and intellectual aspects. Gaining of insight does not always lead to a change in behaviour and it has been said that it means only that the patient has learned to talk about his problems in the therapist's language. This is probably true at the intellectual level of understanding, but it is difficult to believe that the act of translating one way of understanding into another has no effects upon feelings. (See Kelly's Theory of Personal Constructs, Chapter 7).

Faith in the doctor can be as effective a basis for treatment as insight, but even this can be jeopardised if the doctor gets angry when the patient is unable to comprehend the insights he is offered. A simple rule of thumb is that if a patient cannot understand an interpretation it is irrelevant at that point in time. There is a consoling corollary: a doctor can risk making an interpretation of which he is uncertain because if it is irrelevant the patient will not understand it or even apparently hear it. The lesson to be learnt by the doctor is a willingness to bide his time.

Timing

> Mr Followes, aged 38, was a highly-skilled worker, very conscientious and highly thought of by his employer. He was given a job he felt to be beyond him, but he was afraid to say so because his conscientiousness stemmed from

an inability to say 'no' to the demands of people such as his employer; and in any case it was the sort of work he was supposed to be competent to do. He tackled the job, but within a few days his hands broke out in a severe weeping eczema and he consulted the doctor.

'Please get my hands better quickly; I've a terribly important job at work.' The doctor in fact prescribed for him, but had to stop him working, and the certificate was an acceptable reason for the important job not being done. Mr Followes received sick pay and sympathy, rather than the sack he felt he might have received if he had simply said that he was unable to do the job.

It is unlikely that Mr Followes was conscious of a connection between his fears and his eczema. His presentation had the same informative, evocative and promotive structure as Mary Ellard's. The doctor deliberately withheld his interpretation of the symptoms because he did not know how damaging it would be. Instead, he issued a certificate of unfitness, which was quite justifiable, to buy time in which to judge the patient's robustness.

Judgement is also required in deciding whether or not the time is ripe to discover if the patient is deliberately suppressing information or unconsciously repressing it. Looking at the promotive and evocative aspects of his communication often provides the best guide.

Mrs Griggs, aged 30, consulted the doctor very frequently. Her complaints were backache, menorrhagia or amenorrhoea, and vaginal discharge. She seemed to shuffle these complaints and deal the doctor one combination or another without deliberate selection. At no time was the doctor or his consultant colleagues able to find any physical abnormality.

The doctor commented when Mrs Griggs presented with amenorrhoea again that this seemed merely a manifestation of her irregular periods and that to give her tablets to bring on her periods would produce the painful menorrhagia which was one of her alternative complaints. 'Yes, doctor, but when I'm late with a period I'm frightened that I am pregnant.' This answer was more informative than the first complaint, which appeared to have been largely promotive, to get the doctor to give pills to bring the period on and to begin the whole new cycle of complaint.

'If you're frightened that you may be pregnant, I'm surprised that your periods continue to trouble you so much when we can't find anything wrong. I would have thought you would welcome the period even if it was painful.' Mrs Griggs burst into tears. 'My husband doesn't have intercourse with me hardly ever, and he says I'm abnormal in my demands on him.' The doctor was wary of the apparent plea for sympathy and said, 'Are you? What do you do about it?'

There followed an involved story about her having intercourse with other men, after which she would get a discharge or at least worry that she had one, and the whole cycle of complaints would begin again. From this point, some years after Mrs Griggs first presented in the practice, diagnosis was possible and therapy could begin.

When he considered how she had first behaved so promotively, and then made a highly evocative remark about her husband, the

doctor concluded that she must be deliberately suppressing information. He therefore resisted these attempts to influence him and
this brought out the truth.

Often in general practice the doctor is confronted with a patient
who gives him the feeling 'there is something more behind this',
but he is not sure how hard he should push for it at the time. The
advantage of the general practice consultation is that it is unorgan-
ised and unlimited; the lack of formality permits the doctor to play
a waiting game. It is, however, usually necessary to convey this to
the patient, or he will misinterpret the 'waiting game' as noncha-
lance or insensitivity on the part of the doctor. Even doing no more
than this can bring quick results.

> Mrs Hazel was 57, ladylike and a little timid, but the doctor knew from
> past experience that she was able to be firm when she thought it necessary.
> She complained of fatigue, insomnia, anorexia and headaches. 'I suppose I'm
> depressed, doctor, but I can't see why I should be.' 'Well,' said the doctor, 'I
> can give you some pills which will make you feel less depressed, but we won't
> know why you've been depressed. Perhaps it is to do with your not being able
> to discuss things with people, in the same way as you can't talk about your
> depression with me.' 'It could be that,' she said.
> She went on to tell the doctor how her daughter had been living with an
> Indian, was pregnant, and expected her mother to look after the child while
> she went off to India with her lover. She would get married when they were
> established and then send for the child. 'It's so unthinking of her and I
> daren't refuse. She is my daughter, and she will only feel that I am refusing
> because the baby will be coloured—which I must admit I don't like, but then
> I like the illegitimate pregnancy even less.'
> With this opportunity to talk, Mrs Hazel improved and was able to discuss
> the situation with her daughter.

It is neither possible nor necessary to solve every puzzle in communication at the first attempt. Some puzzles can be solved when
more information is acquired, some will never be solved, and some
will go away before they are solved because human beings are
resilient and life moves on.

The undefined approach
This can be considered in terms of listening, questioning and roles.
The importance of understanding the patient's feelings is not just
to make psychiatric diagnoses or to unearth psychological causes
but also to determine how far emotions may be colouring the
patient's account of his symptoms or affecting his comprehension
of the questions he is asked and the advice he is given.

Listening is the basis of understanding. The doctor need not
endure an interminable torrent of words but he does have to stay
alert, relaxed and critical, and it has been shown that there is a

correlation between maintaining eye contact and accuracy in assessing someone's emotional state (Marks et al 1979). He can focus his listening by asking himself how he and the patient are reacting to each other and whether or not any preconceptions he has about the patient are limiting what he hears.

Questions fall into three main categories: *closed*, which demand a very short answer, as in 'Did the headaches start before or after your mother died?'; *open-ended*, as in 'Can you tell me anything more about them?'; and *hidden*, which are statements that invite an answer without insisting on one, as in 'I think you said something about the headaches and your mother's death.' Open-ended questions are particularly useful in the early stages of a consultation because they give the doctor a chance to learn what the patient's assumptions are. They also prevent the patient from being directed too soon by what he thinks the doctor's assumptions are—reading or misreading between the lines of closed questions; and they do not demand the sort of precision in response for lack of which the patient may withold vital information.

The doctor should not try to define his role too soon either. If he presents himself as a father figure the patient may tell him only those things a child could tell a father; if he starts behaving flirtatiously the consultation may never go beyond this level to reach the underlying tragedy. In the other direction, he can never completely determine his own role because some patients will cast his part for him irrevocably before the consultation has ever begun.

Miss Ibbotson, a pretty, flirtatious 19-year-old, whose occasional visits had always provided some light relief in a busy surgery, changed after her marriage into a depressed, rather withdrawn girl, though she was still provocative and flirtatious towards the doctor. Her marriage ended in divorce and only then did the doctor cease to respond to the provocative manner and transpose the consultation to a more serious level. He learnt that she was the youngest child in the family and that her father, to whom she had been attached, had died three years earlier. She still visited his grave regularly and shed tears over it; no man could ever measure up to such a paragon.

Freudian slips

The importance of the revolution in psychiatric thinking which Freud initiated lies not, as is often thought, in the liberation of sex but in the recognition that all behaviour and all speech have a meaning. Slips and errors, lapses of memory and oddities of behaviour, may provide us with vital clues to understanding situations whose deeper meaning may be very different from their surface appearances. On slips and errors, Freud's original work *The Psycho-*

pathology of Everyday Life, is still the best and most entertaining handbook and should be familiar to every practising doctor.

> Mrs Jackson, 26 years old, was attributing her present troubles to an incident in her childhood. On being asked when it had happened, she said 1978 instead of 1968. She had been married in 1978; this was the first indication of any sort she had given that she bitterly regretted her marriage.

Oddities of behaviour as well as speech must be looked at with a discerning eye.

> Mrs Knowles complained of dyspepsia and vague abdominal discomfort and asked for the antacid her previous doctor had prescribed. The doctor's comment that she looked miserable produced a free flow of information about her present difficulties which gave the doctor several opportunities to be helpful. When she got up to go, smiling and grateful, she forgot to pick up the script for which she had come.

A matter of emphasis

A closed question often produces a flat and misleading denial. The strength of the denial can itself be informative but leaves the doctor nowhere to go unless he learns to comment from the feeling evoked in him.

> Miss Long, in her twenties, manageress of her own shop, complained of a never-ending variety of symptoms: aches and pains in various parts of her body, digestive disturbances and many other non-specific ills. Pushed into direct questioning, the doctor received an emphatic denial that there was stress or strain at work, socially, or at home. He confessed that he felt very confused by the variety of her symptoms and by the muddled way she presented them. With a sigh, Miss Long commented that was how she felt about things herself. She was then able to talk about how difficult she was finding it to decide between her career and an offer of marriage.

Symbols

Symbols may sometimes offer a short-cut to understanding but, like metaphors, they have meaning only in context and can rarely be transposed from one culture to another; within a given culture there is no doubt that certain kinds of symbols have consistent meanings and some familiarity with them may be of assistance.

In the following story the boy's unconscious symbolism gave vital diagnostic information in deciding whether or not his abdominal pain might have an organic basis.

> Peter Mason, aged 15 years, had been brought to the doctor or one of his partners several times in the preceding six months with abdominal pains. Appendicectomy had brought no relief and no-one was clear what Peter's symptoms meant. The boy was the only son of a second marriage and had one elder step-brother. Normally a happy-go-lucky sort of boy, he was now getting

depressed by the pains and the failure of many doctors to put him right.

The general practitioner had no success in uncovering any source of unhappiness or conflict until he came to the boy's relationship with his parents. Peter said that they were both kind and affectionate towards him and that he was very fond of them. He went on to remark how good his father was to him; whenever he did anything wrong his father always told him, gently but firmly, what he should have done. This was the first small opening. The doctor commented that it sounded as if the boy felt helpless in the face of authority and that he was getting a picture of a child who never saw any alternative but to submit to what was imposed upon him, however lovingly, by his parents.

The boy denied that he was feeling like this but for the first time showed some emotion, his eyes glistening with tears. The doctor asked him why he was crying and again the boy could give him no explanation, but he did say that he could recall crying like this only once before in his life. It was when he found in the street a woman's purse containing money and handed it over to the headmaster of his school. He remembered how tears had come into his eyes as he did so. It was natural at the time to see that this story symbolised to the boy the way his mother's love, which he valued so much, had always to be submitted to his father's male authority.

The parting words

The tricks of speech that patients have are well worth noting. Such remarks as 'My last doctor said to me . . . ' may reveal much about attitudes and wants, for example. Particularly important are the last words of the patient as he opens the door to go out. This is his last chance before the consultation is over and words may escape in desperation which he had been unable to bring himself to utter earlier on, and he can himself easily escape if they meet with an unfavourable reaction.

Mrs Nettle, who had three young children, paraded each in turn with minor complaints and was obviously dragging out the consultation. When she could prolong it no further and was walking towards the door, she turned and said, 'By the way, doctor, can you get psychiatric treatment on the Health Service?' The doctor took the hint and allowed her to come back and tell him the story of her brother in Scotland who was schizophrenic and of her own fear that, under the stress of looking after her young family, she might go the same way.

Mrs Oakes, in her forties, who had attended the doctor on average once a fortnight for the preceding seven years with a variety of vague complaints, came one evening when the doctor had an empty waiting room. He encouraged her to talk about herself, which she did readily without providing him with any obvious reason for her persistent attendance. When she got up, he felt no more enlightened about the purpose of her regular visits than when she had come. Her last words to him as she went through the door were, 'Thank you very much for your kindness, doctor. Perhaps one day you really will be able to help me.'

The doctor still had a mystery on his hands, but the patient's satisfaction made him wish that he had expressed interest in more direct terms a little earlier, and perhaps saved the need for 150 consultations.

Reference

Marks J, Goldberg D P, Hillier V F 1979 Determinants of the ability of general practitioners to detect psychiatric illness. Psychological Medicine 9: 337–353

5

The doctor's feelings—a sixth sense

Entering the wards for the first time, most medical students are shocked to discover how fragile life is, and how disease, pain and suffering lay waste to it. They are embarrassed to add to their patients' troubles by asking clumsy questions and making even clumsier examinations whose only purpose is to advance their own education. At the same time, they see that the doctors, nurses and other people who are doing something positive for the patients seem not to be impeded by similar emotions. The message to the student is clear: in order to help people it is necessary to become emotionally detached from their suffering. Feeling upset helps nobody. The only useful end that his emotional response can serve is to motivate him to master those skills which offer it a practical outlet.

It is not a very long step from this necessary lesson to believing that to be a good doctor he must pretend, even to himself, that he has no feelings at all, lest he sacrifice his objectivity. Such a belief is utterly misguided and grossly wasteful of a major diagnostic asset. The student is trained in the use of the customary five senses; his feelings can be a sixth sense which, when properly cultivated, can provide him with a great deal of valuable information. Objectivity should govern what he does with it.

No honest general practitioner would deny that his feelings affect his consultations; that, even when they are not caused by the patient who is consulting, they have some bearing on what happens; or that his professional actions are not always guided entirely by expert knowledge and logic. He would certainly have no difficulty in remembering consultations during which he felt anxious, irritated, bored, inadequate, sexually aroused, compassionate, indignant or triumphant, for example.

The most straightforward way of looking at such feelings is to consider how far they are unconnected, indirectly connected or directly connected with the patient who is consulting him.

Unconnected feelings

The doctor's emotional state has an extraneous cause which is usually temporary. He may feel rushed and irritable because he is particularly busy and his car is giving trouble, for example, or he may still be experiencing an emotion aroused by the last patient he saw.

Indirectly connected feelings

One source of such feelings occurs when the doctor has a problem which resembles that of the patient who is consulting him. He too, for instance, may feel incapable of standing up to aggressive younger men, or give in quickly to women who cry in order to get what they want.

Another possibility is that the doctor has a set of habitual responses which, though he is not aware of it, serves to protect him from recognising a neurotic aspect of his personality.

> James Arthur, aged 15, was brought to the surgery by his mother because of acne. When the doctor started to offer his advice Mrs Arthur cut him short. 'I don't want him to be treated here! I want you to send him to the hospital.' The doctor, who prided himself that he was particularly good at managing acne, became angry. The boy was referred. Seven years later he still has acne, is not on speaking terms with his parents, and is frequently in trouble with the police.

In retrospect the doctor realised why he had felt so angry and inadequate in the consultation. He had had acne himself and he had been dragged from doctor to doctor by his mother in an attempt to cure a condition which did not bother him very much. He had been made to do all sorts of bothersome things and to give up foods he liked. He still felt irritated by mothers who imposed themselves in this way on their adolescent sons, and tended to show it. Sometimes a doctor is stimulated into a pattern of behaviour of the kind which is called a Game. This term is defined in Chapter 8 and the ways in which the Games of doctor and patient may interlock are considered in Chapter 9.

Directly connected feelings

The doctor may respond directly to something in or connected with the patient present. He is otherwise relaxed, and no personal problem or Game is involved in his response.

Dealing with the feelings

Because life is never simple, the doctor's feelings may arise from a mixture of the three possibilities, but it is professionally important for him to be able to distinguish between them, at the time if possible, because the ways of dealing with each of them are different. Observation suggests that there are four principal methods: trying to ignore the feelings; explaining them to the patient with some apology; acting them out; and using them constructively.

Trying to ignore the feelings is usually the first response. This seems reasonable enough if the doctor can conceal them successfully and if they are mild enough not to affect his ability to concentrate to any great extent. If he fails to conceal them from the patient he is effectively acting out, whether he is aware of it or not; and, if they are too distracting, he has to put so much effort into trying to ignore them that he misses a great deal of what the patient is saying and doing.

Explaining his feelings and apologising for them is easiest and most obviously appropriate when the doctor knows that his state is both temporary and unconnected with the patient present. He can say, for example, that he is unable to give the proper time and attention to the problem because he has an emergency on his hands, or because he has a bad back—hoping at least that his honesty will be appreciated. Doctors with particularly open personalities may even be able to employ this approach when the feelings are indirectly connected with the patient present: 'I'm sorry, I don't think I can be much use to you because I've got the same problem myself.'

Acting feelings out is a form of communication in itself. It is a truism in medicine that a doctor who gives way to his emotions will be unable to reach a balanced view of his patient's problems, may reward neurotic aspects of the patient's personality and will probably do or say something that he later regrets. Like all truisms, this one is nearly always true, but it does deserve closer scrutiny.

In its milder forms, acting out of feelings is common and not necessarily harmful: looking stern, sounding concerned or being a little flirtatious, for example, can lubricate a consultation considerably. Even when it does not, the patient is not inevitably upset. In more pronounced forms there are two kinds of situation where acting out may achieve useful results occasionally.

A patient who is ashamed or guilty about something he has done may welcome some anger from the doctor, provided that he does not feel totally rejected: it may be easier to bear than prolonged self-punishment.

A patient who finds that his behaviour produces unexpectedly great effects may change as a result. Doctors provoked to anger or sexual interest provide the most obvious examples, but many variations on the same theme are possible.

Miss Buxton, aged 41, had spent the last seven years looking after her elderly parents, one of whom was confined to a wheelchair while the other was becoming increasingly demented. She was being helped by the nursing and social services, but she had almost no life of her own. She visited the doctor from time to time to ask for a small supply of diazepam, to talk, and to cry a little.
Usually he was able to accept his supporting role as having some value, but one day he found himself quite overwhelmed by his inability to do anything more. The way he tore the prescription off the pad and handed it to her must have given his feelings away, for Miss Buxton leaned forward, touched his arm gently, and in a voice full of concern said, 'Don't worry, doctor. I'll get by.'

A doctor who finds that certain patients often cause him to lose his self-control would do better to get a colleague to look after them, and in some circumstances he may need help himself. If acting-out does achieve something useful he can, with hindsight, reckon that he has been lucky.

Using feelings constructively becomes possible when they are directly connected with the patient's manner or situation, and not with problems in the doctor; they can then be very effective aids in diagnosis and management. This is achieved by seeing the patient's ability to provoke the emotion as one of his symptoms: making other people angry (including the doctor), for example, is analagous to having swollen ankles—a phenomenon to be discussed, examined and investigated.

If the doctor can bring himself to think in this way when he recognises feelings rising in him, he will find they subside, leaving him free to think constructively and giving him something new to think about. The patient also has a chance to benefit, since his customary behaviour loses its destructive effects and he is free to explain the real causes of his distress.

Mrs Cummings was a widow of 65. The doctor was beginning to dread her visits because of the way she managed to imply that the intractability of her numerous problems was his fault. He tried hard not to show his irritation and resentment, and generally ended by handing out platitudes and prescriptions. Dissatisfied with this, he decided to tell her what she was doing.
'Mrs Cummings, what is it you want from me? For a long time you've been telling me that nothing I do ever helps you; you don't seem to realise that I'm just like everyone else—I don't like being made to feel useless, and I don't think I'm the cause of your problems. Sometimes it really irritates me, and then I don't even want to try to help you.'
'Ah, so that means you want to see the back of me too, I suppose.'
'There are other people who want to see the back of you, then?'

'Oh yes. My daughter and my sister, they've both turned against me. I don't know why.'
'Do you think they get the same sort of feelings as me?'
'I never thought of it like that. You mean they think I'm blaming them? Perhaps they do. My daughter often says. "For God's sake stop going on at me as though it's my fault."'

This conversation led to a discussion of how she might behave with her daughter and sister in the future, and left the doctor quite pleased with himself and with her. Not all patients can use the insight provided by the doctor's feelings quite as quickly and profitably as Mrs Cummings did, but even so some tension in the consultation may be relieved in a way that improves prospects for the future.

Mr Dodgson, aged 65, consulted the doctor frequently, sullenly complaining of symptoms for which no physical cause could be found. Referring him to hospital evoked politely angry letters from the specialists who saw him. The doctor eventually said, 'I always feel optimistic about getting you better, but I find that I am always disappointed.'
'It's not your fault, doctor, you always try your best.'
'Yes,' said the doctor, 'but it's so unpleasant being continually disappointed that I get annoyed and send you off to another specialist.'
The patient became lively for the first time. 'Yes, that's true, doctor. I feel like that when my back stops me doing a job. My father was always like that: promising me things and then forgetting them or not giving them to me. I used to hate him, but if I got angry when he disappointed me he used to hit me or send me to bed without my supper.'

After this conversation there was no longer any need either to try to conceal feelings or to act them out; the relationship of doctor and patient was better and more honest even though they were no nearer a diagnosis.
Many doctors have difficulty in bringing themselves to try this kind of approach—they think that telling a patient that they have feelings about him is embarrassing and tantamount to admitting that they cannot cope with him. Whether or not it comes over to the patient in that way depends more on the non-verbal cues the doctor gives than on anything else.
Like all techniques, this one is not always appropriate and cannot be used indiscriminately. In some circumstances it may be disastrous for the patient, and in others for the doctor. A patient whose behaviour has left him irretrievably isolated may be worse off if the knowledge is forced on him that he has brought his troubles on himself: projecting the blame on to others may be all that keeps him going. On the other hand a patient whose unpleasant behaviour is bringing him considerable advantages is very unlikely to respond

reflectively to an expression of the doctor's feelings about him, and may well become aggressive. Women who habitually get their own way with men by using sexual provocation present well-known, if rare, dangers of this kind to male doctors.

Feelings that are difficult to use

With Mrs Cummings, the doctor used his feelings of irritation and with Mr Dodgson his feelings of disappointment. These are two comparatively easy kinds of emotions to discuss; others can seem much more difficult. A feeling of depression is hard to admit because in its very nature it reduces the desire for expression; sexual arousal presents the obvious danger of misinterpretation; and anxiety is often concealed because the doctor believes that mentioning it will make the patient more anxious. A few more case histories show that these emotions too can, and should, be used at times.

> Mrs Entwistle, aged 30, was thin, small and miserable. She asked for visits at least once a week for one or other of her three healthy-looking children, and in despairing tones described their incessant coughing or some bout of diarrhoea which it exhausted her to cope with. No amount of reassurance seemed to penetrate her hopelessness.
>
> Very occasionally, just as the doctor was leaving, she would mention that she had vomited or had abdominal pain the day before, and he would say 'If it happens again come to the surgery,' as he made his escape from the depressing atmosphere.
>
> One day Mr Entwistle came to the evening surgery to report that his wife's abdominal pain was very bad and to ask for a bottle of medicine. He did not request a visit and the doctor did not volunteer to make one. A little later the doctor decided that his clinical judgement had been clouded by his feelings about Mrs Entwistle, and that he ought to go round to the house on his way home. He found her jaundiced and suffering from gall-stone colic. She later had a cholecystectomy.

In this case the doctor's feelings caused him to miss a physical illness; if he had been able to mention them the patient might have told him earlier about at least one good reason for her misery. A more common situation is where the patient complains of symptoms that do not seem to have an organic basis, and a depressed feeling in the doctor is the only diagnostic sign to be found.

> Mr Farmer, aged 48, consulted the doctor for the third time in two weeks. He had complained first of backache, but his range of movement had been normal and X-rays had showed nothing unusual; then he had described pains in the chest, neither related to exercise nor accompanied by any physical abnormality. The doctor looked miserably at the record card when the patient made his third approach, but recognised his own reaction. After listening to a description of a rather vague dyspepsia, he led the conversation round to Mr

Farmer's life in general. Some hitherto unmentioned problems emerged, together with symptoms typical of a depression likely to be relieved by antidepressants.

If depressed feelings in the doctor are difficult to use, sexual arousal may present even greater problems.

Amanda Garson, a precocious 16, was attractive and sexually stimulating to the doctor. She complained of loss of appetite, headache and insomnia, reporting them with a bright smile and a show of cleavage. The doctor felt that recognising her effect on him was important, but saw no way in which he could mention it to her. Instead he asked about her boyfriends.

Miss Garson told him vivaciously about the intricacies of her involvement with three young men: it appeared that the one she liked the best was very ardent but never seemed to spend much time with her. This gave the doctor an opening he could take, and projecting his own feelings, he said, 'Perhaps he finds you so attractive that he doesn't know what to do about it?' This drew an immediate response. 'You mean he wouldn't be able to control himself? I feel like that at times. It frightens me when I am really attracted to boys because I want to make love with them so much, and then I can't eat or sleep.'

The doctor's recognition of his feelings had provided him with the key to the problem, and he had been lucky in discovering a suitable way to use them. Without it he would not have been able to do much for her.

Professional anxiety that the patient's symptoms may have a serious cause can arise in a number of consultations. The aphorisms learned as a student are not easily forgotten: 'If you don't put your finger in, you'll put your foot in' and 'Bones are filled, not with marrow, but with black ingratitude; always have an X-ray'. They reduce the doctor's tolerance of uncertainty and tempt him to over-investigate.

Raising the doctor's professional anxiety is a well-established practice of considerable value, and some patients are very good at it. The risk is that he will become resentful when he feels that his anxiety is being raised unnecessarily.

The doctor was called at 11 o'clock one Saturday night by Mrs Hill: 'The baby has been ill for a week and now he can't breathe.' The doctor was far from pleased at receiving a call so late when it could obviously have been made at a more convenient time. He felt even more resentful when he found a happy, apyrexial 13-month-old baby with minimal bronchospasm and three bottles of suitable medicines. The medicines had been prescribed by his partner over the past three weeks. There was no more than one teaspoonful missing from each bottle.

Before the doctor could make any comment Mrs Hill said, 'The baby couldn't take them.' The doctor was tempted to relieve his feelings by demanding 'How do you expect the child to get better if you don't give him his medicine? What sort of a mother are you?' Using his insight instead, he tried a different approach. 'I wonder if you feel anxious because you can't discover what the baby needs and the doctors don't seem to be able to either?'

'Well, what am I supposed to do with him, doctor? He won't take the medicine and I can never get him to eat anything. I get very worried about him.'

Since the baby was obviously in excellent health, making Mrs Hill guilty about not giving it medicine was not going to achieve anything useful.

'Perhaps that's a lot of the trouble,' the doctor said. 'I think we should talk about it when we're both less tired. Never mind the medicines; he won't get worse without them. Come and see me tomorrow.'

The doctor was lucky. Mrs Hill told him some problems the next day which proved comparatively easy to deal with, and the night calls stopped.

Good feelings

A doctor is entitled to enjoy being friendly with his patients, happy that he has been able to help them and pleased with himself when he has done something well. It may seem rather perverse to subject 'good' feelings to the same kind of analysis that we gave to more negative emotions; unfortunately, they do not always imply that everything is well, and they do need looking at too.

There is not usually any desire by the doctor to pretend that good feelings do not exist; it is much more likely that he will show them and act them out. Occasionally, if they have an extraneous cause, he may explain them, but using them constructively can be quite difficult. Admitting what gives us pleasure is in many ways more intimately revealing than admitting the causes of other emotions, and the doctor may well feel that such intimacy is inappropriate in his consultations. It is interesting that the same considerations seem to apply in discussions with colleagues: it is invariably the 'bad' or difficult feelings which get aired in training course sessions devoted to consulting room problems.

Even if the doctor does not want to tell the patient or anyone else about his good feelings, he can acknowledge them to himself and make use of his conclusions. If sexual arousal did not make us feel so guilty, comments about it might have come in this section rather than earlier in the chapter!

The distinction between feelings that are unconnected, indirectly connected and directly connected with the patient present still holds when the feelings are good.

Unconnected feelings

These are unlikely to cause any problems unless they are so strong that they impair the doctor's concentration. Patients note that 'The doctor is in a good mood today', and few who know him will develop unrealistic expectations about his future behaviour.

Indirectly connected feelings

Recognising a problem of his own in one that a patient reveals produces a sense of identification with the patient. If the doctor has resolved his own problem, he may be irritated that the patient cannot do likewise, even with the benefit of the insights or advice that he can offer; on the other hand he may get warm paternal (?maternal) feelings; 'Ah! I remember what that was like,' and feel strong and confident that he knows how to help the patient win through as he did himself.

It is when the doctor has not resolved his own problem that the sense of identification is particularly likely to cause trouble. The glow it brings at first fades in the disappointment of lengthy consultations that lead nowhere, or, as in the story of James Arthur and his mother, the anticipated pleasure of demonstrating special skills is shattered by a patient who believes that someone else can treat him more effectively.

In Chapters 8 and 9 we explain the sort of gains that Games can bring, and describe how a doctor may use his professional position to play them. A Games-playing doctor will be pleased to recognise a patient who will make a suitable partner, and later feels good when he collects his 'pay-off'.

Directly connected feelings

The sense of satisfaction a doctor gets from doing a job well is perfectly legitimate, and it would be altogether too austere not to accept that the feeling will be increased, equally legitimately, if he is thanked sincerely and straightforwardly for his efforts. A small present offered to him in this spirit can be taken with an easy conscience.

Danger lies in the possibility of manipulation, which most commonly takes the form of flattery. It is because we are probably all susceptible to some kind of flattery that the good feelings it produces are considered here as directly, rather than indirectly connected with the patient. So universal a characteristic is difficult to define as a neurosis. Flattery applied cleverly enough is received, at least at the time, as no more than a just recognition of our merits. Few doctors have not at some time been seduced by 'You're the only one who understands, doctor,' for example, and whether the words were heard with pleasure or with resignation, found themselves trying a little harder to 'understand' as a result. It is only when they discover how their professional options have become constrained by their personal desire for the patient to go on seeing them as special, that they appreciate where the temptation has led them.

The doctor who recognises why he felt good initially can use the knowledge in several ways. It shows him why it would be irrational to vent his subsequent frustration on the patient, if nothing more, but it also provides a new base to start from.

The patient's behaviour may be reflected back to him as a 'symptom': 'I get the impression that it's very important to you that I behave in a way you can't get anyone else to behave/I don't do something you're frightened I'll do/I always agree with your point of view'; alternatively a direct confrontation may be attempted: 'Look, I'm afraid this is a bit awkward. You keep on telling me in all sorts of ways what a good doctor I am and that I'm the only person who can help you, and of course that's always flattering to hear. The trouble is that it's made me so careful not to upset you that I've gone along with a number of other things you said and did which I really should have questioned at the time. Now I can't help you at all if I don't start being honest with you.'

If the doctor frequently finds himself a 'victim' in this way, he should suspect that he has an immature or neurotic part of his personality which is leading him into trouble—that his initial good feelings are indirectly rather than directly connected with the patient present, and that he may well be playing a Game of 'Look how hard I tried' or 'I was only trying to help'. To use terms which will be explained later on, he is probably responding with his Child rather than his Adult.

6

Empathy and sympathy

Empathy is defined as putting oneself imaginatively into someone else's position and experiencing the feelings which doing so arouses. It brings an understanding of the other person which makes one less likely to say or do something inappropriate. Sympathy, on the other hand, involves recognising what the other person's feelings are and sharing his view that these feelings are appropriate to the situation.

A doctor who achieves a flash of empathy with a patient remains free to pursue any form of management he thinks right in the light of his understanding; feeling sympathy, on the other hand, determines what he will do. Empathy depends on the doctor's sensitivity and power of imagination, and is always professionally helpful; sympathy depends on his views about life and is valuable only to the extent to which he is right in sharing the view that the patient's feelings are appropriate.

The two stories which follow illustrate the nature and results of empathy.

Mr Abernethy, aged 64, had retired from work when he was 61 in order to look after his bedridden and demanding wife. He came to the surgery only when the district nurse attending her wanted him to get a prescription for dressings, and his visits were always short. The doctor generally asked him in a conversational way how he was keeping, and he would make a little joke about his good health while the doctor was writing out the prescription.

On one such occasion the doctor remarked, without any special thought or reason, 'It wouldn't do for anything to happen to you, would it?' Mr Abernethy said only 'Yes, I suppose so,' but the doctor noticed that he looked down as he said it, and caught an unwonted flatness and hesitation in his voice. It suddenly came to him what Mr Abernethy's life must be like, and for a shocked moment he experienced a despair that had hitherto been hidden from him. He looked more closely and saw the signs of weariness and neglect which he had missed before. Putting his pen down, he got Mr Abernethy to talk about himself for once, and learned how he was beginning to drink quite heavily to keep his thoughts of suicide at bay.

In the next case-history, a moment of empathy taught the doctor how he appeared to the patient.

Robert Black, an immature 17-year-old boy, was brought along by his parents, who said that he had made a sexual advance to a neighbour and that the neighbour had threatened to complain to the police. The parents were very upset. They did not know what attitude to adopt, but were clearly tempted to punish him themselves. The doctor saw Robert alone and, realising that he needed psychiatric help, tried to persuade him to agree.

For a quarter of an hour the boy sat sideways in his chair with his back half-turned to the doctor, answering in monosyllables or not at all, and no headway was made. The doctor then said, 'You are a free agent, Robert, and if you don't want to have anything to do with me that's your privilege. Talking to you now is like talking to a brick wall and there doesn't seem to be any point in going on like this.' For the first time the boy showed some interest and turned to face the doctor, saying 'There is one other thing you can do with a brick wall. You can jump over to the other side.'

The doctor saw the point. From then onward he made it clear that he was on Robert's side of the wall, and not the angry parents', and gained his confidence and co-operation.

Being empathic with many people in a short space of time can be emotionally draining for a doctor to whom it does not come naturally; sympathy is less of a strain, since it is given only when it does come naturally. Both make the patient felt better understood, but the effect of sympathy is to support him in carrying on as he is already doing. The doctor has a status and authority that make his sympathy a more powerful legitimator of the patient's feelings than that of most other people, so that it becomes a professional responsibility to consider whether or not this legitimation is in the patient's best interests.

Mr Coghill was a 67-year-old ex-postman with arthritis in his right hip and both his knees. He lived with his 70-year-old wife who was incontinent of urine and severely disabled by a stroke. He accepted her desire to stay at home, and despite the many services which had been mobilised to help, his life was physically and emotionally stressful. Every month he visited the doctor to collect prescriptions for both of them and would talk for 10 or 15 minutes almost uninterruptedly about the problems he was facing. Then he would leave, thanking the doctor for being so helpful. It seemed that all he wanted was the doctor's recognition and appreciation of his burden; he was not really complaining, in either the medical or the general sense, though his words could have been misinterpreted as complaints. The doctor was entirely in sympathy with Mr Coghill's feeling of weariness, and also with his feeling of pride in carrying on, and this played a useful part in keeping Mr Coghill going.

Recognising the situation not only enabled the doctor to see that his sympathy *was* the treatment, to a great extent, but also prevented him from misinterpreting the complaints as presenting symptoms. Prescribing drugs for everything that Mr Coghill suffered would have achieved nothing, except to cause a rift between them when each drug not unnaturally failed to alter the situation.

Mrs Drabble, aged 29, started her consultation by saying that she was putting on too much weight. Then, crying intermittently, she told the doctor that her husband went out nearly every night and usually came back drunk. His habits at home and his occasional violence frightened her, and were disturbing their 3-year-old daughter. The doctor sympathised with the effect this unhappy situation was having on her. He offered to speak firmly to her husband on her behalf, but Mrs Drabble thought that even suggesting this would make things worse. He then suggested trying some tranquillisers to help her cope, and she accepted them readily. Subsequent consultations followed a similar pattern, and she became a regular taker of the drug.

The status quo, dismal as it may seem, did offer something to both parties. Mrs Drabble enjoyed having someone who was on her side and who confirmed her view of herself as an innocent victim; the doctor enjoyed the feeling of being kind and the warm glow of indignation he experienced on her behalf at her husband's behaviour.

One day the doctor was away and Mrs Drabble was sent in to see a partner. He heard her out in a friendly and courteous way, but he was not at all sympathetic. He asked her how the situation had started and what part she had played in its development. 'Are you saying it's my fault then, doctor? Do you think I want him to be like that?' After repeatedly querying her statements with 'Why?' and 'Is it?', he got a very different story from her. She had married her husband soon after her first fiancé had walked out on her. Her husband knew this and had always felt second-best. It was only after he had found a photograph of the fiancé in one of his wife's drawers that he had started behaving so badly.

On this basis an entirely different kind of management was indicated; preserving the status quo no longer looked like a sensible option.

Sympathy offered too quickly by the doctor can prevent a patient from expressing feelings which are difficult to bring up because they arouse guilt or embarrassment.

Mrs Edwards, a woman of 30, had had two successful pregnancies followed by two spontaneous abortions. She was pregnant for the fifth time when her father, who lived in the same house, died. Soon after this she threatened to abort. The doctor, who had attended both father and daughter throughout, felt very sorry for her and put himself out to show his concern—among other ways by bringing an obstetrician on a domiciliary consultation. The abortion, however, duly took place.

For the next two years the doctor saw no more of Mrs Edwards. When she did return to him complaining of headaches, he saw from her records that she had chosen to consult his partners in the interval, attending with a variety of ill-defined symptoms. The doctor encouraged her to talk, and at length she burst out, 'Don't waste your sympathy on me—I'm not worth it! I've wanted to tell you this for so long. My father was a very difficult man to live with and part of me was glad when he died. And I didn't want to hold on to that pregnancy either. But I felt so bad about it I couldn't possibly tell you when you were being so kind and sympathetic.'

Sympathy is a very specific kind of management, with definite indications and contra-indications. It should be used only when the doctor has understood the nature of the problem he is treating, and only when he believes that its known effects will be of benefit. As with any other treatment, the rationale requires review from time to time.

When we looked at empathy we noted that it might have a cost to the doctor, if he found it emotionally draining; the cost of sympathy is paid by the patient if he loses the opportunity to develop and mature. Part of the bill for sympathy is also footed by the NHS if the general practitioner expresses it with prescriptions, investigations or referrals that are unnecessary on clinical grounds. Referral can lead to unnecessary investigations and operations by specialists, and given the scope of modern medical technology the cost of inappropriate sympathy may be very high in financial terms.

The 'sympathetic approach'

The conclusions we have reached about sympathy may seem to be at odds with the everyday usage of the term, in which a 'sympathetic approach' is always good. This approach consists of being friendly, courteous and relaxed, but it does not require the doctor to share, as our more precise definition did, the view that the patient's feelings are appropriate to his situation. The problem of trying to use ordinary words in a special way is, as usual, insuperable.

However imprecise, the term 'sympathetic approach' does suggest a way of behaving that is clinically valuable. We can define it as trying to understand the feelings which underlie the patient's behaviour rather than reacting directly to the behaviour. To friendliness, relaxation and courtesy this adds the desire to be as objective as possible; it may not be 'sympathetic', strictly speaking, but it is an approach which we can recognise and work towards. The careful listening which it demands is always appreciated and may sometimes be therapeutic in itself.

Mrs Franks was a woman of 40, well-known to all three partners in the practice. She was a frequent attender at the surgery with complaints that mainly concerned her lower abdomen. No kind of therapy had ever made any difference. On one of her visits the surgery happened to be very quiet and the doctor encouraged her to tell him about herself and her early life.

Mrs Franks disclosed that her father and mother had separated when she was 2 years old, after which she and her mother had lived with a harsh and forbidding aunt. Her childhood was unhappy; and when she was 17 she fell pregnant. The baby was adopted, and four years later she got married.

The next year her mother died of carcinoma of the cervix, and she mentioned that memories of this always came back to her when she saw any blood. Her husband was a kind and understanding man, but she was always so tense, and attacks of panic overwhelmed her so often, that she felt she must be very tiresome to live with.

The doctor said that anyone would agree that her life had been unfortunate and that he could see why she worried about being tiresome to live with, but he made no attempt at interpretation, and Mrs Franks departed. In the succeeding year she consulted him only three times, and then with complaints which were amenable to therapy. They were on much better terms when they met and each of the consultations seemed to satisfy both of them.

A 'sympathetic approach' may not always produce quite such obvious benefits to both patient and doctor, but making one has obvious effects on their relationship, and in our present state of ignorance we can remark only that this is in some way healing.

7

Fostering a relationship

In each relationship a person makes he reveals something about himself, and, if there is a common theme in all his relationships, it must have a connection with something fundamental in his personality. The doctor-patient relationship therefore gives a doctor the opportunity and the means to study his patients' personalities and to understand the contexts of their illnesses.

At times it may do even more than this. The patient who can make a relationship with his doctor of a kind that he has never had before may learn from this experience how to transform his relationships with other people. When this happens, the relationship is not just an aid to diagnosis—it may be said to have a therapeutic use as well.

> Mrs Childs, aged 24, was in bed with the curtains drawn when the doctor visited her. She was complaining of nausea, a severe headache and photophobia, and when he examined her the doctor found that she had a temperature of 102.2°F, a pulse-rate of 62, definite neck stiffness and an equivocal Kernig's sign. He diagnosed meningo-encephalitis and explained to Mrs Childs why she would have to be admitted to hospital. He was not at all prepared for the reply: she flatly refused to go.

The doctor had done what he had been taught to do. He had explored and evaluated his patient's problem, explained his findings and offered his expert advice. This sequence had served him well while the problem was the physical illness, but he felt less confident that it would do so when the new problem appeared.

> 'What makes you not want to go into hospital?' he asked. Mrs Childs looked petulant. 'I've had a lot of trouble at the hospital in the last two years. I just don't want any more.'

At this juncture we can retire from her bedroom to consider the three sources of information a doctor relies on to guide his clinical actions. For the sake of brevity we can call them the Traditional, the Continuing Personal, and the Here and Now, and imagine them as levels at which different kinds of information are stored and awaiting integration.

The Traditional source is the sea of medical knowledge in which all general practitioners cruise. The medical and surgical specialities are dotted about in it like islands; few patients know how poorly it is charted, or how frequently the doctor is out of sight of land.

The Continuing Personal holds information that the doctor has gathered from his previous contacts with the patient, only a little of which is to be found in the medical records. The patient has Continuing Personal knowledge about the doctor too; it is from this level that each derives many of the expectations that he has about the other.

The Here and Now is new for every consultation, and often the best way to explore it is to pose the questions Why this? Why today? and Why me?

The consultation with Mrs Childs illustrates the value of the Traditional approach—it led the doctor to his diagnosis and told him what advice he should give; but its limitations are exposed as well. How can he use the other two levels?

> Mrs Childs's notes showed that before registering with the practice six months earlier she had had two episodes of cystitis, followed by an appendicectomy at which an acute right salpingitis had been found. She had continued to complain to the doctor's partner of RIF pain and lethargy, and had been referred to a gynaecologist at the local hospital. After giving her a course of antibiotics, the gynaecologist had written 'I think there is a tendency for this patient to become introspective about her gynaecological state of health and I think we must try to discourage this'—a few faint clues for the Continuing Personal file, but not enough to work on.

The doctor had noticed on entering the Childs' house that though it was beautifully furnished, it looked unlived in. Mrs Childs had seemed extraordinarily calm when she complained of her blinding headache; her refusal to be admitted to hospital had reminded him of the response of an obstinate child. The doctor thought he had a fresh clue to explore in the Here and Now which might illuminate her reason for refusing admission to hospital.

> 'Have you any children?' he asked. Mrs Childs burst into tears. Mr Childs, her husband, had let the doctor in, looked on anxiously throughout the consultation and supported her in her refusal to enter hospital. Now he said 'We're very worried about it; in fact we have a private appointment with a new gynaecologist tomorrow.' The doctor suggested that if Mrs Childs would go into hospital he would explain to the new gynaecologist why they were breaking their appointment. 'We can talk about it when you come out.' Mr Childs smiled with relief, his wife's face lost the look of obstinate petulance; the doctor arranged admission to hospital.

The crisis was over; the doctor's work, however, had hardly begun. He now had the beginnings of a Continuing Personal file. 'Mrs Childs, a pretty woman with meningo-encephalitis, has a good-looking and caring husband, a well-cared for house, and no children. She has had gynaecological problems. She appears withdrawn. She looks obstinate and petulant when confronted with a situation which she cannot control.' The doctor's evaluation (perhaps guess would be a better description) at this stage was that Mrs Childs had probably been depressed for some time; that her husband encouraged her petulant behaviour when she was thwarted, possibly because he was frightened by it: and that there might be problems about sexuality as well as gynaecology. He wondered how good a mother a petulant child would make.

One way in which the doctor can test his understanding is to make predictions. In this case, the doctor predicted that Mrs Childs would become petulant whenever she was thwarted. He decided that, for the immediate future, he would avoid disagreeing with her as long as this was safe, though he would try to make it clear that he was not frightened of confronting her. In effect, he transferred his rather scanty information from the Here and Now level to his Continuing Personal file and used it to plan his own future behaviour. The long-term goal was still to help Mrs Childs manage her own relationships better.

After she had recovered from her illness, Mrs Childs told the doctor that intercourse with her husband had been frequent until the attack of salpingitis had left her with dyspareunia. She spoke with little emotion. When a fresh appointment with the gynaecologist was discussed, she gave a smile when she said 'I hope you don't feel that we're forcing you into this,' but there was no warmth in it. 'Not if it's what you want.' the doctor replied, although he did feel forced and was not enjoying carrying out his plan. He added to his Personal Continuing file the observation that Mrs Childs was aware of other people's feelings, but that she was not affected by them.

The gynaecologist found no reason why Mrs Childs should not become pregnant. Mrs Childs said she was pleased, though no signs of pleasure appeared on her face. She sat with ankles neatly crossed, gloved hands clutching each other and leaning forward a little, looking for all the world like a well-behaved child at an interview with the head teacher.

'We do so want a baby, but my husband works terribly hard and he's away on business so often. Couldn't you get him to take me with him? I'm sure I'd get pregnant if we went away together.' The doctor wondered why she needed him to put the point. 'I wouldn't have thought you'd have much difficulty in persuading him yourself, but you can certainly say I think it's a good idea. Would you rather I told him?' 'No, I think I'll tell him myself. Thank you very much.'

The doctor thought he had taken a small step forward by showing that he was willing to let her use him even though he was aware of what she was doing.

Mrs Childs became pregnant. Sharing her care with the hospital, the doctor felt that his relationship with her became more intimate. She showed her emotions when she talked, and she showered him with questions about preparing for the baby. He answered them, but knew that sooner or later he would have to ask her why she was not putting them to her mother or to her friends.

His information at the Continuing Personal level was growing slowly, and he began to see her as someone who never had an acceptable model of how an adult should behave. This might account for her behaving like a petulant child. Their relationship did not yet seem strong enough for him to say this to her; it still needed fostering.

After a normal delivery, Mrs Childs became a radiant mother, and her face was far from expressionless when she handled the baby. She asked to be fitted with a cap, and continued to ply him with naive questions. The doctor judged that the time was ripe to move forward. 'Didn't you have the opportunity to learn that from your mother?' he asked, in response to one of her questions. Mrs Childs's face froze. She gathered up the baby like a parcel and made to leave.

The doctor backed off. 'I've upset you,' he said.

Mrs Childs's face unfroze a little. 'I don't suppose you meant to,' she said. 'I'm a little touchy today. My husband is away again. I've not been sleeping. Could I have some sleeping tablets, do you think?'

The general practitioner returned to his original plan.

'Well, I'm a little unhappy about that. Mightn't you sleep too deeply to hear the baby if she woke up?'

For the first time in many consultations Mrs Childs looked petulant again. 'I really do think I should have the sleeping tablets,' she said. The doctor had strong views about prescribing sedatives in such situations. 'I'm sorry, but I really can't see my way to prescribing them for you,' he said. Mrs Childs looked increasingly sulky and the doctor felt somehow trapped. 'Surely you can manage without?' he suggested. Mrs Childs left looking sullen, with the doctor feeling that his plan had suffered a major setback.

Four days later Mrs Childs came by herself to the surgery to see him. She sat down, took a deep breath and began to talk at great speed.

'I've got to tell you. You've always known, haven't you? I've got to tell you or you won't be able to help me.' There was no sign of petulance.

'What am I supposed to have known?'

'I'm full of hate. I've always been full of hate. I don't want to be full of hate. It's awful. I love my baby so much. I don't want to go on with this hate inside me. It's not my fault. It was the way of my childhood. I'm not really to blame.'

She carried on describing how she saw her life and the way that people had treated her, and it was a remarkably fluent presentation. She told the doctor that her father had been 40 when he married, and her mother 18. He was wealthy and she was pretty. 'I suppose it was his last chance to get a young girl, and she married him for his money.' Her father travelled a lot. They had been living in America when Mrs Childs was born, and when they came back to England her father had been arrested and put in prison. 'I suppose that is how he got his money.' she said. She had felt close to her father before his arrest.

Almost immediately after this her mother took in a man called Bill to live with her. 'I hated Bill,' said Mrs Childs. 'I still hate him. He was the beginning of my hating.' Her father came out of prison when Mrs Childs was 8 years old. There was a row, Bill left, and the marriage was resumed. 'Prison did something awful to my father.' said Mrs Childs. 'He became a dirty old man.' She described how he was constantly trying to see her undressed, how he had offered her money to take her knickers off, and how, when she was older, he tried to pay her and her pubescent friends to let him 'feel them'. 'He even tried to have intercourse with me, and when I refused he called me ugly and went on calling me ugly. I hated him. My mother knew and didn't do anything to stop him. I hated her too. Of course, she was going out with Bill again.'

When Mrs Childs was 16, her mother left home to go and live with Bill. Mrs Childs felt she couldn't stay with her father. She left home and school, where she was about to take 'O' levels, and got a job. She never saw her father again, and he died a couple of years later. 'I was glad,' she said. 'I hated him!'

Her mother's mother then gave her a home, and for the next two years she helped nurse her grandfather, who was dying of cancer. Her mother never visited her father when he was dying. When her grandfather died, her grandmother was found to have cancer too.

'Then', said Mrs Childs with heavy emphasis, 'then my mother and Bill moved in. They were living with their two children in a caravan and they only came so they could get grandma's house. But they didn't. I was so glad. I hated them so much, my mother and Bill. I couldn't stay in the house even though my grandmother was so ill and I loved her so much. I left and got a job in London. I never saw my grandmother again and she died about a year later. I hated myself, but I couldn't go back while my mother and Bill were there. When I heard Grandma was dead, I tried to commit suicide, but I was too much of a coward.'

She had met her husband shortly after. 'I married him because he was strong and because I knew he would make money. I didn't love him. I do now, but I hate myself for not having loved him before.'

The end or the beginning

For the first time in nearly two years of a relationship which he had tried hard to foster, the doctor felt he had a reasonably complete Continuing Personal file. He believed that the information available at all three levels had been explored and that he could now evaluate it. He had an explanation for Mrs Childs's behaviour in their consultations and he felt justified in his assumption that her behaviour with him reflected what was happening in her other relationships. His plan for fostering their relationship seemed to have been justified; they would now have to wait and see whether her sudden confession had brought her any lasting benefit.

There is a tendency for doctors to believe that when patients unburden themselves the work is over; in truth it may just be starting. Nevertheless, if a relationship has been built which the patient believes is strong enough to test with intense and intimate information like that given by Mrs Childs, the hope that it can be used therapeutically is a reasonable one.

We have seen how the doctor observed Mrs Childs's behaviour and used his interpretation of it to anticipate the difficulties he might meet in developing a relationship with her. Her behaviour and her interpretation of other people's behaviour seemed to be highly idiosyncratic and he recognised that he would have to take some risks if they were to reach a common understanding of her problems. The harrowing story eventually elicited makes it easy to understand how Mrs Childs came to place constructions upon behaviour and relationships which differ sharply from those in common use.

All human beings try to make sense of the world around them. Kelly's Theory of Personal Constructs (Kelly 1965) offers perceptions about how people do this which can be usefully applied within the doctor-patient relationship. Like most theorists, Kelly uses words with special meanings and invents new terms—they are described fully in *Inquiring Man* (Bannister & Fransella 1971). Kelly's fundamental postulate sees human beings as active explorers of the world around them, testing the 'sense' they make of reality by using it to predict future events. This Kelly calls 'construing' reality—or creating 'constructs': a construct identifies certain things or themes as similar yet different. Kelly illustrates this by taking the construct 'black versus white', which is relevant in terms of shirts, shoes and paper, but irrelevant in terms of affection for children or the distance one lives from one's surgery. The construct can be used to describe a patient's skin, which is appropriate in some contexts and inappropriate in others. As well as being 'appropriate versus inappropriate', constructs can be 'similar versus dissimilar', so that a shirt a son calls 'white' (versus black) might be called by his mother 'black' (versus white). All constructs are bipolar, but it is possible for two people to have constructs which share one pole but not the other: one person may construe food as 'tasty versus sour' and the other as 'tasty versus sweet'. Each of us has a personal system of interrelated constructs, the components of which we select by their usefulness in interpreting and anticipating events: we may be blind to logical incompatibilities in our own system if recognising the illogicality would disturb the way we want to see things. Mrs Childs's constructs for interpreting relationships appear to have included 'mother versus trust', 'trust versus hate' and 'compliance versus anger'. For the doctor to help Mrs Childs it was essential for him to identify these constructs so that he would, as Kelly puts it, 'play a role in social processes' which involved her. Perhaps this was what Mrs Childs meant when she opened her cathartic statement with 'You've always known, haven't you?'

Exploring someone else's construct system is often seen as aggressive. The hostility it provokes is an avoidance response to an attempt to make a person examine attitudes which are rooted in feeling rather than logic. This is probably why Mrs Childs reacted with such hostility when the doctor questioned her about learning from her mother; it also probably explains why many doctors are wary of confronting patients in too stark a manner with any illogicalities in their personal system of constructs, Mrs Childs's catharsis could have resulted from her recognising that, in the light of her own motherhood and her new experience of mother-love, she had to change some of her most important constructs.

The logic of Kelly's theory is elegant and attractive. Its usefulness to any doctor will depend upon the extent to which it helps him construe the events he observes and anticipate developments in his relationships with patients.

References

Kelly G A 1955 A theory of personality—the Psychology of Personal Constructs. W W Norton & Co, New York
Bannister D, Fransella F 1971 Inquiring man—the theory of personal constructs. Penguin Education, Harmondsworth

8

Dishonest relationships

An honest relationship suggests that the parties to it have a common view about its purpose, will tell each other everything that this purpose demands and will not use it to pursue covert purposes of their own. What does this mean in the context of the doctor-patient relationship in general practice?

The first two propositions clearly need special consideration. Doctor and patient may not take the same view about the kind of relationship which is necessary for the purpose of helping the latter attain the best state of health possible. In a widely-quoted paper, Szasz & Hollender (1956) discussed three possibilities, each having an appropriate place: doctor active and patient passive; doctor guiding and patient co-operating; and mutual participation. A doctor who believes that no other options are acceptable will be uncomfortable with a patient who believes it is perfectly proper to have a passive doctor and an active patient, or a doctor who co-operates while the patient guides. How else can we explain the irritation of a doctor when a patient comes in and announces that he needs an X-ray?

Perhaps the doctor wants the patient to complain of a persistent cough or shortness or breath, and to admit that he smokes 20 cigarettes a day, upon which cues he will recommend a chest X-ray himself. Perhaps a sensible patient learns to adapt to this view even though he does not share it. The result may be a charade, but since all relationships have to allow for idiosyncracies of the parties involved, calling it dishonest is too strong a reaction.

It is generally accepted that a patient will tell the truth about himself, apart from those minor lies which are necessary to keep the relationship flowing smoothly, though what he says will be constrained both by what he thinks is relevant and by what he prefers to conceal. The doctor can influence both constraints—the first by the sort of questions he asks and the second by the trust he engenders—but it is the patient's right to withhold any information he chooses without being called dishonest, as long as he accepts the consequences of doing so.

Total honesty is not generally expected of doctors, though some patients are less willing than others to let the doctor do their thinking for them.

The first two propositions may leave room for discussion; the third does not. When either party describes himself or his situation in ways that he knows to be untrue, or pretends to emotions that he does not feel in order to pursue purposes that remain covert, the relationship becomes dishonest. It is not always the case that the other party is deceived: sometimes he takes care to avoid recognising the deception, and sometimes it is unimportant to him because he had a dishonest purpose of his own. A doctor-patient relationship which is dishonest is most unlikely to be therapeutic.

A patient may be trying dishonestly to obtain some material benefit or drug which requires the doctor's signature, or to enlist his support in struggles being waged in his family or elsewhere. The doctor may be taken in; he may refrain from probing too deeply because learning the truth would leave him with some awkward choices, including calling the patient a liar; or he may ignore the available clues because he is busy with a dishonest purpose of his own, pretending that he is more concerned and caring than is really the case, for example.

A doctor may start being dishonest because he wants to persuade a patient to follow a piece of advice he knows would be resisted if he told the truth, to avoid difficult discussions, or because he does not care enough about the patient to give the extra time that honesty would require. The patient may be taken in; he may refrain from probing too deeply because learning the truth would leave him with some awkward choices, including calling the doctor a liar or a coward; or he may be too busy trying to create a false impression— that he is already doing everything possible to deal with the problem he is presenting, for example.

A special kind of dishonest relationship, where at least one and usually each of the parties is being dishonest with himself about the purpose of the interaction, has been described by an American psychiatrist called Eric Berne. His work on the theory and practice of Games appeared first in 1961 in the book *Transactional Analysis in Psychotherapy* and again in 1966 in the best-seller *Games People Play*.

GAMES ANALYSIS

A pattern of behaviour can be called a Game if it fulfils three strict criteria:

— it is repeated by the 'player' frequently enough for there to be a legitimate suspicion that it serves some important purpose, however obscure

— it evokes from another person responses which the player can then blame for his own situation, allowing him to avoid accepting responsibility himself

— the manipulation of the other person is not deliberate and conscious. If it were, the player would lose the gains he is after, because knowing that their origin was dishonest would make them worthless. The pattern of behaviour is learned early in life, with the player's parents as teachers, and is developed pragmatically without the player being aware of it.

The dishonesty, albeit unconscious, of using another person to satisfy unacknowledged needs is clear enough, but Berne goes further. He says that a player will not be able to involve another person in his Game unless that other person wants to play a Game of his own: there is always a way of declining an invitation. The seasoned player rarely has difficulty in finding a partner to play with.

A doctor may recognise Games in his patients' behaviour in the course of taking a history; he may witness them being played by a husband and wife who are being seen together, for example; or he may realise that a patient is playing a Game with him during a consultation.

From what was said above, it should follow that a patient will be able to play Games with a doctor only if the doctor wants to play a Game of his own. This is not entirely true in a professional relationship, since some Games can be declined only by walking away. As long as the doctor has a legal and moral responsibility to find out if his patient is ill, he is not free to take this action. Nevertheless, Games-playing doctors are not uncommon, and the situations which arise when doctor and patient play together will be discussed in the next chapter. The rest of this chapter will be devoted to saying a little more about Games Analysis and to describe a few of the Games which a general practitioner is likely to hear about or witness most frequently in the course of his work.

Use of the term 'Game' does not imply that what is at issue is trivial, or of entertainment value only. Berne was thinking of the conflict involved, the opportunity to win, and the rules which determine the actions of the players. Some of the Games defined can be played with an intensity that results in litigation, injury or even death.

The purpose of every Game is essentially defensive: someone who feels inferior or inadequate plays Games which allow him to judge others as being no better than himself; someone who feels guilty will choose Games that make him feel blameless; someone who sees himself as weak will go for Games that prove the other players to be ungrateful—and so on. Good Games have social advantages too, but their psychological strength lies in their power to protect the player from having to do anything constructive; they defend the dismal 'position' of the player's deepest fears about himself. Only when this is understood can the observer make sense of the player's habit of putting himself over and over again into situations where the people he chooses to spend his time with turn out to be ungrateful, unhelpful or unsympathetic with unfailing regularity. The value of Games Analysis lies in the way it makes clear the point of patterns of behaviour which may otherwise be baffling. The stories which follow illustrate a few of the many Games which have been described.

'Why don't you ... yes but'

Mr Anthony, aged 42, was overweight and beginning to get short of breath on exertion. Angina and ischaemic heart disease were common in his family. In his medical records a partner had commented that the patient took no notice of the advice offered to him and that she had referred him to an out-patient clinic because he insisted that his condition needed complicated hospital tests. After attending the clinic, Mr Anthony told his general practitioner that the appointment had been a waste of time. The specialist had not ordered many tests; seeing the dietician would mean taking time off work which might cost him his job, and diets were too expensive anyway; his beer-drinking, which was not heavier than anyone else's, was necessary to replace fluid lost by sweating, and giving it up would destroy his standing with this mates; he knew he could not give up smoking because he had tried unsuccessfully many times. His ECG was said to be normal, but one of his brothers had been told the same thing a few months before he dropped dead of a coronary. His wife's efforts to help by changing the menu were a waste of time because her cooking was now unpalatable and unsatisfying.

The Game called 'Why don't you ... yes but' proves to the player that other people are no cleverer than he is—no matter how exalted their status. He can always show that the suggestions they make for the problem he poses are incompetent, impractical or illogical, and he is pleased rather than dismayed as he does so. Their failure is his 'pay-off', since it confirms his 'position'. If not even the experts have a good answer, there is clearly no point in trying to do anything himself. The only way in which another person can avoid giving him his pay-off is to decline to play, with a response like 'That's a very difficult problem. What are you going to do about it?'

Games bring social as well as psychological gains, as 'Why don't you . . . yes but' illustrates clearly. Someone whose problem defies even the experts can not only forgive himself for doing nothing about it, but can expect others to forgive him too. He can also take a leading part in the sort of conversations which go on in pubs and trains about how useless experts are.

'Wooden Leg'

Mr Braden, aged 31, visited the doctor soon after moving into the area of the practice. He said he needed sleeping tablets quite frequently, because his nerves were so awful, and complained that no-one understood how hard it was to have such an affliction. In the factory where he worked, his prospects depended either on doing a physically hazardous job or on taking supervisory responsibilities; either option was impossible to contemplate. His wife was annoyed with him because he had shouldered none of the problems of moving house, though he had been the one who wanted to move. All he desired was a quiet life, which was not much to ask. His nerves had been 'terrible' for as long as he could remember, so he supposed he must have been born with them. If blind and deaf people had allowances made for them, he deserved some equivalent dispensation. Perhaps the doctor could at least make his wife understand this.

The name of this Game is short for 'What do you expect of a man with a wooden leg?' The all-important disability may be epilepsy, alcoholism, a stammer, angina or anything else that can be used as an excuse for evading social and personal obligations. It allows the player to be free of blame and to get sympathy from casual acquaintances, and it wards off the depression which honest self-appraisal would provoke. To decline an invitation to play, the other person can reply 'I don't expect anything. What do you expect of yourself?' and if he is a doctor he should insist on an answer within a reasonable time. The story of Mrs Drabble (Chapter 6), who received inappropriate sympathy from one doctor, but was later helped by an unsympathetic partner, can be interpreted as an illustration of the handling of a Game of 'Wooden Leg' where the disability was 'a brute of a husband'.

'Psychiatry'

One variant of 'Wooden Leg' which will be familiar to all general practitioners goes by the name of 'Psychiatry'. It does not rely simply on 'terrible nerves' as an excuse, but uses the language of psychiatry itself to provide irreproachable reasons for a player's behaviour.

Mrs Corrigan, aged 34, sat herself down in the consulting room, clasped her knees to her chest, and delivered the following monologue: 'You don't know me, because I'm actually a patient of one of your partners who is away on holiday. I'm being treated at the psychiatric clinic for a psychosomatic bowel complaint—I get diarrhoea whenever I have an exacerbation of my anxiety state. Last week I had a row with my employer as a result of a rather ridiculous communication failure, and my colon reacted immediately. On Sunday night I phoned the duty doctor, but he refused to come out. My husband was angry, started projecting his hostility on to me, and I developed such a tension headache that I wasn't able to keep my appointment at the psychiatric clinic on Tuesday. I knew that my own doctor was away, but when I saw the psychiatrist on Friday he said that my emotional reaction was quite predictable, and that was reassuring. Now I've lost my job, but my condition is settling because the psychiatrist gave me some tablets to sedate the intestine. All I need is a certificate backdated to when I first suffered my reaction.'

Anyone can pick up enough jargon to play this Game, but the skilled exponent serves his apprenticeship in the many clinics to which he is referred, where he is not so much looking to be cured as learning how to be a better neurotic. Since the defence is expressed in terms of diseases from which the player claims to suffer, the only way of countering it is to display a degree of scepticism about how valid these are as excuses. It is easier to push him back to his underlying 'Wooden Leg' and employ the usual antithesis to that.

'See what you made me do'/'Harried'

Mrs Dunstable, aged 39, came to the surgery complaining of pains in her arms and legs, but within a few minutes began to speak of more personal matters. She was deeply upset because her mother had just died, and she would have liked some support from her husband. He was too wrapped up in his own interests to provide it, and, as she put it 'He's never been any help really, doctor! He always wants me to make the decisions about everything.' If she ever invaded his privacy to ask his opinion, she would be met with abuse for interrupting him at a crucial moment and making him do something wrong, but if her decisions turned out badly, he would be furious about any disturbance that was caused to him. Rows of this sort were now almost the only kind of communication she had with him. She did not expect him to change, but his selfishness in her present distress was making her so much worse that she was crying all the time.

The doctor offered to see her and her husband together and, rather to his surprise, they both kept the appointment. Mr Dunstable put his point of view with some hostility. His wife had always liked to organise everything, and to make her happy he had let her do so. He complained only when she did something particularly stupid, which was quite often for someone who had such a high opinion of herself. The present outburst of hers was ridiculous, and based on just one incident: she had started crying just when he had to go out for an important appointment and he had been annoyed with her for making him late.

At this point Mrs Dunstable burst into tears. Mr Dunstable rolled his eyes to heaven and said 'That's how it is. I don't think this coming to the surgery's been a particularly good idea. We'll have a performance all night now, and I'm supposed to be up very early tomorrow.'

The doctor felt more sympathy with Mrs Dunstable than with her husband, but realised that she must have been acquiescing in his behaviour throughout the 12 years they had been married. Perhaps she was playing a Game of her own. Mr Dunstable's attempts to absolve himself from blame and cope with feeling pushed around ('See what you made me do') could have been countered early on by leaving some of the decisions up to him, but she had opted instead to play 'Harried', a Game in which the player takes on far more responsibilities than he or she can cope with, and this had provided an excellent excuse for failing to discharge any of them.

This case shows how Games interlock. The husband and wife each allowed the other to feel free from blame when things went wrong, so that neither would want to alter the pattern. Only when some outside event came along and changed the priorities of one of them would there be a cry of 'Foul!' In some marriages the tension set up by interlocking Games like these has the effect of making sexual intimacy pretty rare. Husband and wife may both see this as a further advantage.

STRUCTURAL ANALYSIS

Underpinning his work on Games, Berne created a discipline that he called Structural Analysis. In this he proposed that there are three readily identifiable states in which the personality of every individual, regardless of age, can be seen to function. He named them the Parent, the Adult and the Child, and at any one time, one of these ego states will be in control of a person's behaviour.

The Adult is the state in which we function rationally and plan how to cope with the problems of everyday life. The Child is the primitive, spontaneous state; it is in charge when we are being creative and when we are responding instinctively to constraints imposed upon us. The Parent directs us when we react in either the nurturing or controlling ways that we perceived in our real parents when we were children. Each of these states is valuable and necessary at certain times, but when we function in a state that is inappropriate to the situation, our behaviour may be described as neurotic in some way.

An example may make this clearer. Suppose a man says to his

wife 'Where is my tie?' She may answer in three ways. If she says 'It's on the bed,' her Adult is speaking; if she says 'I didn't move it. Why ask me?' her Child is in control; and if she replies 'If you didn't always leave things lying around you'd be able to find them when you want them,' it is her Parental state that has been evoked.

The Parent and the Adult will be out of place when we are having fun; the Parent and the Child will get in the way when we need to work out our priorities in a complicated situation; but we will need the qualities of our Parent when we are responsible for the well-being of someone who is incapable of looking after himself.

Structural Analysis looks at a person's behaviour in terms of which ego state is in control at any point in a transaction with someone else, and its implications for clinical consultations are obvious.

> Mrs Edmonds was known to the doctor only casually. A brisk 40-year-old woman, she consulted him to say: 'I don't think you know, doctor, but I have had a radical mastectomy. I know it was for cancer and I know what I'm supposed to look for. I've just found a small lump in my left armpit, and I think I should see the surgeon earlier than has been arranged.'

The doctor was somewhat taken aback by this rational presentation. When he examined her he found things just as she had said. She was functioning in her Adult mode, and though this was appropriate for the circumstances, her behaviour was unusual in the doctor's experience.

> Mrs Farquhar, a 40-year-old multipara, had had a hysterectomy a few months earlier. She had lost 42 pounds in weight when the surgeon made this a condition of the operation, but she was now back to 224 pounds. She said she wanted to diet again because her husband found her unattractive. The doctor reminded her that she had been trying and failing for years, and that she had even regained the weight she had lost pre-operatively. 'I know pills don't help me, doctor, and I know I break my diet. Perhaps if I came to see you every week to be weighed I'd really be able to lose weight.'

Her words were sensible enough, but it did sound as though she was talking about a difficult child. In Structural Analysis terms, her Adult was asking the doctor to help in controlling the impulsive workings of her Child.

> Mrs Grantly, aged 60, had never consulted the doctor about an emotional problem before, and he thought of her as a thoroughly sensible person. She complained of feeling anxious and of what she called nervous dypepsia. 'I'm very upset because the house next door to us has been bought by Indians, and everyone knows how dirty they are. We can't afford to move now that my husband has retired.' It transpired that she had no personal experience of Indians and knew no one who did, but she was unwilling to look at the situation rationally.

Irrational statements of this sort, often pompous and traditional, come from the Parent. Any attempt to debate them calmly with the Adult is likely to meet with Parental anger.

> Mr and Mrs Hildren, a couple in their late twenties, came together to the doctor to complain that their 15-month-old daughter would not sleep properly at night, and either cried for hours or came into their bedroom. In discussing the situation, it became apparent that any remark of the doctor's which could be construed as sympathy for the parents was welcomed, but suggestions that they might be a little more tolerant of the child seemed to come against a brick wall.

The doctor thought that his Parent was being invited to help control the baby, and that he would satisfy the Hildrens only if he acted accordingly. His professional Adult opinion would not interest them.

Little dramas of this kind take place in every consulting session, and their real meaning is rather different from what appears to be going on at the Adult level. When thought of in terms of Structural Analysis they can be recognised quite easily: the anxious mother whose Child is seeking reassurance from the doctor's Parent for example, the angry father whose Parent wants the support of the doctor's Parent, and the flirt whose Child brings out the Child in the doctor. Appreciating that consultations are not always transactions between the Adults of doctor and patient is an important step that Berne made it easy for us to take.

Structural Analysis also allows for conscious dishonesty in a relationship, with what are called 'ulterior transactions'. These always involve three or more ego states, unlike simple transactions between one ego state on each side. One kind of ulterior transaction is illustrated by the exchange:

Salesman: This one is better, but you can't afford it.
Housewife: That's the one I'll take.

The salesman's Adult makes two objective statements that appear to be directed to the housewife's Adult. If her Adult had made the reply it would be to say that he was correct on both counts, but, as he expected, he hooked her Child and got the answer he wanted.

Another kind of ulterior transaction is typical of flirtations:

Cowboy: Come and see the barn.
Female visitor: I've always loved barns since I was a little girl.

At the social level this conversation takes place between their two Adults, but at the psychological level there is a sexual invitation from the Child of the cowboy to the Child of the visitor, and a sexual response from her Child to him.

Mrs Ives, aged 32, was a plump and pretty woman with two sons whose health she fussed over rather ineffectually. She was heading for obesity like her mother and consulted the doctor spasmodically to discuss the minutiae of diets to which she never adhered. When she brought the boys to the surgery one day with the usual snuffly colds, the doctor decided to try a different approach. He looked her up and down slowly, then said 'It really is a shame you have such trouble losing weight. You'd be extremely attractive if you were just a bit slimmer!' Mrs Ives blushed deeply, said something akin to the Restoration Comedy phrase 'La! doctor!' and proceeded to lose three stone in the next three months. She came to the surgery regularly to show off the progress she was making—each time wearing a different expensive new outfit—and stopped bringing her sons. The doctor wondered what her husband thought about the cost of her metamorphosis and put the question delicately to her. The answer came with a smile and another blush: 'Oh, I earn the money myself—I always have. Anyway, he loves it—he can't keep his hands off me!'

The doctor's new approach could be taken as coming from his Adult and addressed to hers, but it was obviously heard by her Child, as he expected, and showed her how she could please him. How far it is permissible to pursue a professional purpose by non-professional methods, and whether she felt that it was his nurturing Parent or his sexual Child that was speaking, are both open to debate. There can be no doubt that the transaction was decidedly ulterior!

Structural Analysis is not only a study in its own right and the basis of Games Analysis, it is also the foundation of Script Analysis, an outline of which is given in Chapter 10.

9

Playing Games with the doctor

In the last chapter we noted that players become skilful at recognising people who will accept their invitations in order to play an interlocking Game of their own. There are some Games, however, which can be avoided only by walking away, and a doctor who is unable to do this because of his professional responsibilities may therefore become involved in them unwillingly. One Game of this sort is called 'Kick me'.

'Kick me'

> Mrs Ackroyd, aged 40, was a patient whose very name produced groans from everyone in the practice. The sequence of events to be described was pretty typical of the way she behaved.
>
> One Wednesday evening at 11.30 pm she phoned the partner on call and told him that her 7-year-old daughter Gloria had a terrible cold and was sneezing so much that she could not go to sleep. The doctor offered to see Gloria in the surgery the next morning and advised her that an immediate visit was unnecessary. Mrs Ackroyd did not bring her daughter in on Thursday morning, but at 10 pm she phoned the same doctor to say that Gloria was no better and that she was getting very worried. The doctor's reply did not conceal his annoyance.
>
> On Friday Mrs Ackroyd brought Gloria to the surgery and consulted a different partner, whose irritation when he heard the story was not reduced by finding Gloria to be no more that slightly snuffly. He brushed aside the mother's requests for a note for the hospital and an X-ray, and propelled her from the room with a prescription for a linctus.
>
> On Saturday night a request for a visit was made to a third partner in terms of such urgency that he had to go. When Gloria was found to be asleep and certainly no worse, the doctor was unequivocally angry. Just what did Mrs Ackroyd expect him to do? 'I don't know why you're so annoyed, doctor! I never trouble the doctor unless someone is really ill, but all I ever get is abuse. She's been bad for a week now, and she hasn't had any treatment for it. It's the same thing every time, and now you're going on at me! You do nothing, then you pick on me!'

'Kick me' is a Game played from a position of low self-esteem through which the player invariably gets confirmation of his belief that other people try to kick him around. The apparent plea 'Don't kick me' inevitably brings the opposite response if the demands are

70

unreasonable enough, and the player then collects his 'pay-off'. Doctors are not always unwilling victims, though. Sometimes they have Games of their own and recognise the chance to play them with patients who have suitably interlocking Games. In Chapter 5 we classified situations like these as ones where the doctor's feelings were indirectly connected with the patient present.

'I'm only trying to help'

This is probably the Game most commonly played by people in the 'caring professions', like doctors and social workers. When anyone's best efforts to help are spurned or criticised, he is entitled to feel a little aggrieved—the hall-mark of the Games player is that this happens to him repeatedly.

The outcome reinforces his belief that people are ungrateful, and this enables him to avoid the unpleasant feelings of weakness and inadequacy which characterise his 'position'.

A doctor's Game of 'I'm only trying to help' interlocks beautifully with many Games played by patients. The pairing with 'Why don't you . . . Yes but' is particularly obvious because his efforts are rejected so quickly; with 'See what you made me do' the rejection takes a little longer. Most Games-playing patients make suitable partners because they are not truly looking for medical help at all, only a chance to collect a 'pay-off'.

> Miss Ballard, aged 29, had an odd habit: she would consult any of the doctors in the practice with her problems initially, but for the follow-up she always went to one particular partner. She would complain to him about some aspect of the first consultation, or its outcome, with an air of injured innocence which he found irresistible, and he would protest on her behalf to whoever was responsible—the partner, the doctor in an out-patient department or someone in the town hall, perhaps. Almost always he received a reasonable explanation, and if Miss Ballard's reports were less than honest it was a tribute to her influence over him that he found himself in the same situation so often. He did try one or twice to get her to confess to some exaggeration, but desisted when she put on an expression which indicated that he had let her down by not being forceful enough. None of the episodes had a proper conclusion: each ended only when she stopped coming back about it, and when she had a new problem she would start by seeing a different partner again.

Miss Ballard was playing 'Let's you and him fight', classically a Game for women, with male partners. It seems to indicate a desire to express contempt and probably masks some sexual fear, but to the outside observer the effect is rather comic. Miss Ballard had identified the partner who could best be relied on to give her her 'pay-off': he was the one most susceptible to her charms and also the one most keen to get his own 'pay-off' from 'I'm only trying to help'.

Just as a doctor is constrained to become an unwilling partner in a patient's Game when his professional responsibilities prevent him from walking away, so a patient who is reluctant to default from treatment can find himself involuntarily involved with a Game-playing doctor. There is an aggressive Game called 'Now I've got you, you son of a bitch' which can easily be adapted to the clinical situation by a doctor who wants to justify his 'position' that people are not to be trusted. The player seizes on some minor wrongdoing of the other person and makes a wholly disproportionate issue out of it. So, a doctor who frequently makes remarks like 'Well, you've only got yourself to blame. If you'd taken all the tablets/stayed flat on your back/kept your appointment/come to see me earlier and not gone to a quack, you wouldn't be in this position. There's nothing I can do now,' gives grounds for suspicion that he is playing such a Game.

The patient who partners him need not be so innocent—'Kick me' and the closely related 'Why does this always happen to me?' both interlock well with 'Now I've got you'. Presumably it is only patients who want to play Games like these who persist in consulting such an unpleasant doctor. Others, unless they are obsessional enough to behave perfectly, will find their way to a different doctor.

Finally in our illustration of Games played with the doctor we should not forget the interlocking Games that provide a quick 'pay-off' to both parties in the shape of good feelings, the potential danger of which we have looked at in Chapter 8. Berne delightfully called them 'Gee, you're wonderful, Dr Murgatroyd' and 'My, how uncommonly perceptive you are'.

Analysing Games is something more than a diversion for doctors who enjoy the exercise. It offers a new range of diagnoses and also methods of management that are derived logically from understanding what is going on.

Diagnosis

The value of putting a name to a patient's condition is that we can refer to a body of accumulated medical knowledge for ideas about what to look for, the causes that may be at work, the outcome that may be expected and the form that intervention should take. In this respect, psychiatry is not as advanced as, say, cardiology, and there are times when it can be difficult to distinguish a psychiatric diagnosis from an insult.

In the case-histories quoted in this chapter and the last one, what is the name of the condition of the obese Mr Anthony, the lazy, neurotic Mr Braden, the selfish Mr Dunstable, the bossy Mrs Dunstable, the demanding Mrs Ackroyd and the seductive Miss Ballard? In fact the name of the Game that each one plays has almost all the characteristics that we required of a diagnosis—a behavioural diagnosis perhaps, but then it is the patient's behaviour which is in question. We can also enjoy the relief which being able to apply a label brings in its own rights.

In the early stages it may be difficult for the doctor to recognise a Game because of the way that he is involved in it himself. When it becomes clear what the Game is, he will have a better understanding of what is going on, an idea of what to look for, the possibility of making predictions and some thoughts about the courses of action that are open to him.

Eight responses

Having diagnosed the Game, there are eight possible responses that the doctor can make.

The first is to ignore the dishonesty he has recognised, because his need for the 'pay-off' of his own Game is greater than his need for professional self-respect.

The second is to become a partner unwillingly because he cannot walk away. At least he knows why he is going to lose!

The third is to become a partner deliberately and consciously, either out of compassion or to gather evidence which he hopes to be able to use later on.

The fourth is to try to get the patient to play a different Game— one that at least has temporarily more useful effects.

> Mrs Churchill, aged 76, had been taking to her bed over several months, and was now staying there all day. She tried to get the doctor to sanction this with a mixture of 'Gee, you're wonderful, Dr Murgatroyd' and 'Wooden Leg', but he concluded after examining her that the risks of activity were less than those of becoming bedridden. Realising that reassuring her about her heart would produce only more symptoms and more flattery, he chose instead to pour scorn on malingerers and rebuke her for wasting his time. She then opted for 'I'll show him' as a way of getting a 'pay-off', and within a fortnight was up all day.

The fifth is to decline the invitation, and the pseudo-medical request that goes with it, but giving no explanation for doing so even when there is a vigorous reaction. The patient usually then looks for a more amenable doctor, but if this is impracticable he is likely to become depressed.

The sixth is for the doctor to set rules within which he will accept the demands that go with the Game. 'You can have 20 tablets a month but under no circumstances will you get any more,' or 'Since telling me about your problems seems to help you, we can set aside 15 minutes ever fortnight specially for that. I'm afraid I can't offer you any more.'

The seventh is to show the patient the nature of the Game he is playing, hoping that in time he will be able to discuss ways of behaving differently. Again there is a strong possibility that the patient may become depressed, as he is deprived of his defence against self-understanding.

The eighth is to teach the patient about Games Analysis as a pre-liminary to discussing the Game or Games that he plays.

Of these alternatives, the first three allow the doctor-patient relationship to continue, though each has a different aim; the fourth tries to use it to bring about a temporary improvement; while the last four put it at risk, in one way or another, in the hope of pro-ducing a more lasting benefit. Understanding Games enables the doctor to decide which of the last seven alternatives is most appro-priate to the circumstances, and should make him aware of any tendency he may have to pick the dishonest one.

The depression which may occur when his Game is refused must be seen as the first step in the patient's recovery and be treated on its merits.

10

Scripts

We all know someone who seems to make the same mistakes over and over again, or to follow a self-destructive path that he is unable to abandon. He may make many marriages, for example, all of them similarly unsuitable; he may be 'his own worst enemy' in turning on anyone who could or would help him; or he may make a habit of running away when anyone gets too close to him.

Our inability to understand people like this makes any relationship with them difficult; and, very relevant in the consulting room, our inability to influence them makes it likely that we will end by rejecting them. To find some way round this unhelpful state of affairs Berne and his colleagues developed an approach to behaviour patterns of this kind which they called 'Script Analysis'; focussing as it does on the patient's whole life-story it should be of particular interest in general practice.

This short chapter offers a brief and highly simplified outline of Script Analysis; the best introduction to the theory and how it is derived from Structural Analysis (Chapter 8) is given in Berne's book *What do you say after you say hello?*

SCRIPT ANALYSIS

A Script is a programme which an individual constructs in early life under parental influence; it is usually completely written by the time he is 6 years old, and it directs his subsequent behaviour in the most important aspects of his life. Presumably everyone receives some programming, but not everyone appears to follow it rigidly over many decades. Script theory takes this into account, though it is not yet well enough developed to be able to estimate the frequency with which people learn to depart from their scripts, or at what stages of their lives they do so. 'Scripty' behaviour is most easily recognised in its extreme forms, and poses a difficult challenge to the general practitioner who meets it.

Berne describes certain elements which can be discerned in the apparatus of a Script. Three of them make up the Controls: a Curse, an Injunction and a Come-on; four provide ways of combatting the Controls: a Spell-breaker, a Permission, a Demon and a Counterscript: and one, Parental Behaviour Patterns, can serve either the Script or the Counterscript. These unusual terms require some explanation.

The Curse is a message conveyed to a child by his parents from an early age, and hammered home by constant repetition: 'You'll end up like your father!' or 'With your temper you'll kill somebody one day!' Curses differ in detail, but all are variants of one of four themes: 'Be a loner'; 'Be a failure'; 'Go crazy'; and 'Drop dead'. In Structural terms, the Curse comes from the Controlling Parent of the mother or father, and is incorporated in the child's Parent.

The Injunction is a warning, also repeated frequently to the young child; and transgressions are punished. Some Injunctions are mild ('Don't be too ambitious') and failure to heed them provokes nothing much worse than disapproval. Tougher ones, like 'Don't answer back!', 'Don't you dare tell your father!' or 'Don't get too attached to anyone!', are backed up by emotional blackmail or even by threats of physical violence. Insofar as boys especially want to please their mothers, and girls their fathers, an Injunction which comes from the parent of the opposite sex is particularly powerful.

The Come-on. In a normal family, a child tries to please his parents and is rewarded by a feeling of closeness and a sense of security when he succeeds. There are parents, however, who do not give this reward readily, so that the child is made anxious and forced to behave in ways that do not come naturally to him to win their approval.

Such a parent may seem to do nothing worse than say things in company which put the child at a disadvantage or embarrass him ('John will have the last cream cake—won't you, John?') but even this has powerful effects if it is done frequently and consistently. In more extreme cases the parent may sneer at the child maliciously. Whatever the level of pressure, the child's insecurity motivates him to succumb to the temptation of the 'See if you can please me' message from his destructive parent.

In the terminology of Structural Analysis, this temptation is the voice of the parent's Demon, whispering to the child's Demon. As the child grows up, the parent's voice is incorporated into his own Parent, and from within him goes on whispering to the Demon in his Child, egging him on to acts of which he is ashamed or which may even destroy him. It says 'Go on, have another drink!' or 'Now's your chance!', and he is conditioned not to resist. A Control of this sort is called a 'Come-on' and any Script that contains one will be a loser's Script.

The Spell-breaker provides a condition which, when satisfied, lifts the Injunction, and frees a person from his Script. The condition may relate either to time ('After you pass the age at which your father died') or to an event ('After you have had three children'). It comes from the parent's Child to the child's Child. To help someone escape from his Script, the therapist has to find out if there is a Spell-breaker, and what it says.

Permissions. Parents impose the restraints in a child's Script Controls, but they may also give him Permissions—to enjoy himself, to do things well or to be able to drink in moderation, for instance. Permissions do not operate autoimtically as Controls do, but when a person invokes them they allow him to behave adaptively. The more Permissions he has, the less tightly bound he is to his Script.

The Demon is that element of the personality which is totally unpredictable—the most primitive and autonomous part of the Child. It can defeat both the strictest Controls and also the best efforts of the therapist to lift them.

The Counterscript. This is the sort of well-meaning maxim by which a father or mother tries to influence the values of an older child, typically in his teens. Examples include 'Save your money!', 'Work hard!', 'Keep your head!' and 'Never draw to an inside straight!' Advice like this does not have the same power as a Control, but if it opposes the message of the Script there is a chance that reinforcing it may be beneficial. It comes from a parent's Nurturing Parent and is incorporated in the child's Parent.

A Counterscript influences a person's life-style while his Script controls his destiny: a Devoted Housewife may make the newspapers as Mother of the Year or when she Leaps from Roof of Tower Block. Berne tells of a girl whose father's Curse was 'Drop dead' and whose mother added the Counterscript 'Never go in the wet without your wellingtons,' She was dutifully wearing them when she jumped off the bridge.

Parental Behaviour Patterns. While the Injunction usually comes from the parent of the opposite sex, the way of behaving on which a child models himself is most often that of the parent of the same sex. Like the Counterscript, Parental Behaviour Patterns exert their main influence on the older child. They come from the parent's Adult and are incorporated in the child's Adult.

Not all Scripts are loser's Scripts : some are programmes for winners. A winner's Script will contain a Blessing rather than a

Curse ('Be a great man!') or an Injunction that is adaptive ('Don't be selfish!'). The Come-on will be replaced by 'Well done!', the Spell-breaker may be readily available, the Permissions may be plentiful or the Counterscript helpful. With these kinds of good luck, and as long as his Demon remains friendly, a winner's Adult will be in charge of his life and he will set his own goals.

Winners say things like 'I made a mistake but now I know what to do,' losers tend to say 'If only . . . ' In between them are the non-winners, who see the bright side of losing and say 'Well, at least I didn't . . . '; they are people who cause little trouble and make good employees.

A person's Script tells him who he is and where he is going; it therefore determines which Games he will play by marking out the 'position' from which he plays them. This concept was taken further by other colleagues of Berne, who described four basic positions that a person can adopt in his relationship with other people:

I'm O K—You're O K:	the healthy position of winners
I'm O K —You're not O K:	the position of arrogant mediocrities; clinically paranoid
I'm not O K—You're O K:	socially self-abasing and psychologically depressive, this is a loser's position
I'm not O K—You're not O K:	the position of those losers for whom everything is futile; clinically schizoid or schizophrenic

The case-history which follows is different from any other in this book because it does not describe events in which one of the authors was involved. It is a modified version of a story recorded by Berne, chosen for its simplicity and for the clear way in which it reveals many of the elements of a Script apparatus.

Mr John Appleyard went to the doctor, partly at the instigation of his wife, complaining of tiredness and insomnia. He was 49 years old, with four children, and worked inordinately long hours as a sales representative on commission. He was a heavy smoker, and had a blood pressure of 180/110 as well as marital problems. His father, a compulsive worker too, had suffered a coronary thrombosis in his fifties and been forced to retire prematurely. The patient recognised that he was following in his father's footsteps, and knew where they led; he said that his financial commitments left him no option, though he had made a few half-hearted attempts to change his job.

The doctor had a strong impression that Mr Appleyard was tightly controlled by a Script, and when they analysed the patient's life for evidence they found plenty of it.

The patient was an only child. He had been very close to his mother, and his father had frequently been away from home, working. He clearly recalled his mother telling him when he was little 'Remember, in this world you mustn't ever give up, even if it kills you!' From his father he had learned the way to obey this Injunction, and it looked as though the result was a Curse which condemned him to death. Both his parents had exhorted him in his teens to work hard. The only saving grace came from his father in the form of a Spell-breaker: 'You can relax when you have a coronary.'

This meant that it would be no use warning him that his way of life might bring on a heart-attack. Not only did he know this—he actually needed a 'coronary' to free him from his Script, and he could think of nothing other than a breakdown in his health that would do this for him. The doctor's aim, therefore, was to convince him that he could relax before having his coronary by giving him the necessary Permission.

At first Mr Appleyard's only understanding of his situation was that he was trapped in a way that frustrated, angered, and depressed him, but after a few consultations he began to see the nature of the forces that had trapped him. His wife was present at these consultations, and she lent her own support to the Permission which the doctor gave. Mr Appleyard then managed to find another job, at rather lower pay, in the offices of a local charity, and also took on some private book-keeping as an extra source of income. He still worked hard, but the blind compulsion disappeared, and at the age of 50 he was free to be his own man for the first time in his life.

In the terminology of Structural Analysis, Mr Appleyard's Child had received the Injunction from his mother and the Spell-breaker from his father; his Parent had been given the same Counterscript by both of them, which reinforced the Script; and his Adult had learned about how to work hard from his father. The Permission strengthened the aspirations of his Adult and Child to be free, though his Parent ensured that he would continue to be a hard worker even in his new life.

Other therapeutic approaches, using other terms, could perhaps have achieved the same result, but the strength of Script Analysis is the way it made clear so quickly that it was a Permission that was required, rather than advice about slowing down, or an explanation of the reasons why the patient was working himself to death. This indicated to the doctor that he must aim for the kind of relationship that would enable him to provide it—one which made Mr Appleyard regard him as extremely powerful.

It is worth noting that Permission in Script Analysis does not mean exactly the same thing as the permission we refer to in the syndrome 'Permission to get better' (Chapter 12) a static situation in which a patient carries on having symptoms unnecessarily after his illness has been cured.

In Chapter 8 we commented that Games Analysis at least offered the doctor a way of making sense of baffling behaviour, even when he could do nothing about it, and at best gave him a rational basis for treatment. It may not be too optimistic to suggest that Script Analysis has similar possibilities for the general practitioner.

11

Happy and unhappy families

There seem to be two extremes of behaviour by families in relation to medical help. At one extreme are the families whose members seem unable to help one another and are always turning to outside agencies for aid, freely discussing absent members and demonstrating their own and each other's incompetence, and never seeming to cope without the doctor's intervention.

At the other extreme is the family which is very tightly knit and gives the doctor the feeling that he is always an outsider, useful for specific purposes but never brought into the family circle. Troubles are never exhibited to outsiders until they erupt in public: a court case, a divorce, an illegitimate pregnancy or something which can no longer be concealed and which, when brought to the doctor's notice, takes him by surprise. Help is usually possible only after the crisis has occurred.

With the first type of family it is all too easy for the doctor to respond to the authority with which he is invested by usurping roles which should be filled by family members. He then not only fails to gain understanding, let alone show it, but may increase the difficulties posed by the amorphous nature of the bonds within the family to an extent which can be catastrophic.

> The doctor was called to Mrs Arliss who had just moved into the district and found her in labour at full-term. Her husband was not in the house and there seemed to have been no preparation at all for the birth. The doctor arranged for Mrs Arliss' admission to hospital and for her two small children to be cared for temporarily by another patient who lived next door. He managed to contact Mr Arliss and also to set up a variety of supporting domiciliary services.
>
> He was frequently consulted about the rearing of the child and went out of his way to give psychotherapeutic help to the woman during her next pregnancy, which was unwanted. He met the husband only occasionally over minor ailments and never within a family context. Over the next two years the woman consulted him more and more often with her four children. He should not have been surprised when she came to tell him that her husband had begun to go out with another woman.

This may have been unavoidable, but the doctor had surely undertaken responsibilities which properly the husband should have met. He had also missed an opportunity, which the time spent on Mrs Arliss during her pregnancies might have afforded, to find out whether or not her husband wished to be more involved. With families who exclude him the doctor may have no alternative but to wait.

Antenatal care of Mrs Box in her first pregnancy revealed evidence of emotional problems but the doctor's attempts to elucidate them met a brick wall. She had difficulty in rearing her child, having frequent recourse to the well-baby clinic and later to the ordinary surgery. Simultaneously her husband began to consult the doctor about dyspepsia for which no organic cause was found. Still the doctor could not get either partner to accept any connection between their individual difficulties. He felt excluded and irritated. Within three years the woman appeared in the surgery in great distress with an extra-marital pregnancy.

This eruption of intra-family difficulties may also have been unavoidable, but the omens had been obvious enough, and when all the doctor's overtures were rejected his failure was perhaps that he did not discuss this exclusion with the couple.

The hierachy of elders
In a static society one generation can draw on the experience of another to help bring up the children. Our society is too mobile geographically and socially for this always to happen, and its mores change so rapidly that the experience may not be useful when it is available.

Many of the functions of well-baby clinics and health visitors are recognisable as ones that an educated elder relative might fulfil. The paradox is that if the doctor gives instructions about the early part of a child's unbringing without a proper understanding of the effects of his intervention on the family development, he may increase, rather than diminish, later developmental problems.

The doctor was called out one evening to a 3-month-old firstborn child. The story of a miserable child crying in pain was borne out by first appearances, but not by his examination, and the child quietened as he held him on his own lap for examination. Still holding the baby he tried to explain to the anxious mother that it was her anxiety and uncertainty which exaggerated the state of the child. The father nodded wisely during the lecture. Mrs Candless looked relieved that the child was no longer crying. The doctor left well-satisfied, but the mother's resentment of this demonstration of her incompetence damaged his relationship with her irrevocably, and soon afterwards the family transferred to another doctor.

Only a hair's breadth separates acceptable advice and the demonstration of incompetence and it is difficult indeed for the doctor to resist the temptation to show the mother or the father how to do the job and so finish up doing it rather than explaining it.

Sparing the child

Parents have to learn that some trauma is necessary for a child's development and that every child is entitled to love. The single-child families of the 1930s produced a widespread fear of 'spoiling' children, not understanding that an only child suffers from a surfeit not of love but of anxiety. A major swing occurred after the Second World War as Dr Spock's first book caught the imagination of American and British parents, and permissiveness ruled. Now the pendulum has begun to swing back and parents are likely to be advised to provide some regularity for their infants and not necessarily allow the caprices of their children to rule the household. These swings of fashion cause problems because parents are encouraged to bring up their children in ways which differ from those in which they were raised themselves and the implied criticism of their own parents may be difficult for them to take.

> The doctor was called out late to a 15-month-old firstborn child. The dramatic history of inconsolable crying was belied by the happy child who was sitting in mother's arms. Full examination revealed only sore gums and erupting teeth. Mrs Derby said, 'I know he's teething, he's cried the last few nights and we have taken him to bed with us like my mother suggested. It stops him crying but it stops us sleeping and we're both becoming exhausted.' The doctor suggested that it was quite permissible to pick up the baby, give him a mild analgesic as well as a cuddle and then put him back to settle in his cot. The parents both gave a sigh of relief.

In the case of Mrs Candless the doctor had demonstrated his competence and the mother's incompetence, producing effects which were not predictable because his action was undertaken with insufficient family knowledge. With Mrs Derby he was dealing with nothing more than the problem created by the culture lag of modern folk medicine. He made a common-sense statement which was in effect a therapeutic trial and which, had it failed, would have told him that he needed to examine the family situation in more detail.

Common sense can make uncommonly onerous demands on people asked to show it; the doctor should think carefully before making such demands.

> Mrs Everly, the mother of two healthy boys, could never accept the inevitability of their occasional respiratory infections nor her own inability to prevent them. When the doctor realised this, he questioned her gently and

learned that her sister was in a mental hospital and that she had fears about her own adequacy and mental stability.

Persistent demands upon the 'common sense' of Mrs Everly before the doctor knew these details, were doomed not only to fail but possible also to cause damage. It could be said that we are making of doctors the common-sense demand that they make a diagnosis of why a person appears unable to be commonsensical.

Mrs Forrester continually brought her 5-year-old son to the doctor seemingly unable to tolerate the slightest cough or coryza. The doctor asked if she had had similar difficulties with her firstborn son who was now 20. It emerged that she had had no difficulty in rearing him, but the second conception had been unwelcome and she had attempted to rid herself of it. She still felt guilty and was constantly looking for weaknesses in the child whom she felt she had injured before he was born.

Inherited confusion

The 'parent in the head'

Parental influence remains for ever. Just as in every fat man there is said to be a thin man trying to get out, so in every emotional difficulty there is a 'parent in the head' trying to make its influence felt—an idea obviously related to Berne's Structural Analysis (Chapter 8).

Mrs Glazier, a patient new to the doctor, asked him for tranquillisers. She kept losing her temper with her 9-year-old daughter and got into such a state that she had to walk for miles before she regained control. The doctor asked her about her relationship with her own mother and was told that her mother was kind and gentle and never had to raise her voice. 'What is your mother saying inside your head now?' asked the doctor. The woman replied, 'Don't let her get on top of you, my girl!' A picture rapidly emerged of a rigidly domineering mother who could quell with a look and of the patient vacillating between the permissive attitude she had adopted towards her own daughter and an acute anxiety that the latter would turn out to be as uncontrollable as her grandmother.

A young woman, Mrs Harlan, complained of her second child's failure to become 'dry' by the age of two years. This child was a girl; the first had been a boy. Whilst she talked the child poked head and fingers inquisitively into everything in the consulting room. The mother kept saying placidly, 'No! Don't do that!' The child took no notice whatsoever. 'What is your mother saying in your head?' asked the doctor. 'Watch out or she'll be the boss!' was the immediate answer. 'What's your dad saying?' 'Just the same thing!' was the reply. 'Why don't you want to listen to them?' asked the doctor. 'Because it's no fun being a child who has to obey all kinds of rules she doesn't understand.'

In this last case we can hear not only the 'parent in the head' but the whole family story. That childhood memories should affect one's relationships with one's own children is readily understandable, but their effect extends to all personal relationships.

> Mrs Idle complained that she was unable to relax during intercourse, and was always nagging her husband just like her mother had done to her father. The doctor asked what her father was saying all the time in her head. She replied without hesitation, 'You horrid little child!'

> Victor Jobling, aged 19, complained of being on the verge of a nervous breakdown. Clarified, this meant that he consciously feared he was a homosexual. His main anxiety was an awareness of a wish to avoid women, rather than being positively attracted to men. When asked what his father was saying inside his head he thought for a moment and said, 'Nothing, he has no time for me.' Asked what his mother was saying he replied, 'Do as I want and I'll be nice to you.' He then went on rapidly to describe how domineering she had been and how she had used him in her endless battles with her husband.

From these stories it will be seen that patients are often aware of the 'parent inside the head' and will answer what, on the surface, seems a very odd question. Once the door was opened the patients readily discussed the intrusion of past parental authority into their present life.

Roles and relationships

General practitioners doctor families because families live together. Whether illness is familial, hereditary or environmental, families share illnesses and individual illnesses affect other members of the family. Thinking of the family in terms of Roles can be helpful. A role, in this meaning, is a set of behaviours which the family needs to have filled if it is to function. When a family member becomes unable to fill a role the balance of the family changes and its ability to survive will depend upon the flexibility and viability of the bonds which exist between its members.

The scapegoat

In any disordered family relationship it will be found that a particular situation evokes a set of attitudes in each member towards each other member, which none seems able to change even when it is glaringly inappropriate. A vivid example is the creation of a 'scapegoat' on whom all the guilt is heaped, thereby strengthening the bond between the others, reducing their guilt feelings towards each other, and rendering their misdeeds mere peccadilloes by comparison with the evil behaviour of the black sheep.

> A 12-year-old boy, the eldest of four children, was brought because his school reports said he did not try and spent his time clowning. Mrs Kent, his mother spoke bitterly, 'My other three do so well, you would think they

would shame Kenneth into doing better.' The doctor had, however, seen the situation develop over the years. He remembered Kenneth complaining that his father had never been interested in anything he did. The father had been a neglected only child and his bonds of sympathy with others were weak. Kenneth had begun by striving for approval, but finding little reward had then adopted his father's attitude of indifference, and finally turned in despair to clowning to get attention. As this happened the three other children grew up comfortably under the umbrella of Kenneth's misdeeds and even the bonds between husband and wife were strengthened as they struggled to cope with such a difficult child.

Whilst it is usually a child who is the scapegoat, it may be a parent.

Mrs Law, a woman with teenage children, said she felt on the edge of a breakdown. For years she had caused occasional upsets in the family, with both her husband and her children, but she was doing this so frequently that even the children were saying 'What shall we do with our problem child?' The doctor knew the husband to be a deeply disturbed narcissistic character, who maintained his own precarious health by manoeuvring his wife into these outbursts, and pinning on her the label of 'ill member', which he himself would have been unable to wear without breakdown.

The management of disordered family relationships

We have highlighted the danger of the doctor's unthinking entry into a family situation, taking on a role not really his. Many disordered family relationships stem from the neurotic inability of one member to play his proper part. The temptation for the doctor is to attempt to correct the situation by giving his diagnosis and issuing instructions.

Young Mrs Morris brought her 7-month-old baby to the doctor, complaining that he had began to cry in the night and requesting something to make him sleep. The doctor noted that teeth were beginning to erupt, and discussed the baby's great need at that stage for parental proximity and love. The mother returned a few weeks later saying that the baby was no better. This time the doctor saw how she sat with her baby on the end of her knee with a foot of space between him and her own body. He tried to make her hold the baby more securely and warmly, but even under instruction the mother seemed unable or unwilling to cuddle him. She did not consult that doctor again, but a year later was still haunting the surgery requesting sedatives from his partners for a baby who would not sleep.

In this case again the doctor was confronted with a woman telling him that she was frightened to love her baby, and instructing her to do so could only increase her anxiety; they both knew that she was incapable of demonstrating love at that time. If instead he had attempted to evoke the maternal side of her that was being inhibited, he might have made a small start towards helping her with her difficulties. Contrast this with the following case.

Mrs Narovic was a gaunt, formidable woman from Eastern Europe in her forties. She brought her 12-year-old girl, as she had done many times, to complain that the child did not eat, had no energy and frequently had abdominal pain. Anna had been investigated at two different hospitals, with no abnormality being found, but the mother insisted that a third hospital must be tried. 'Look at her, pale and skinny; she must be ill!' Indeed the child, curled up on a chair crying, looked a pitiful object deserving of her mother's contempt. It was obviously useless to try rational reassurance again, and while the mother went on talking the doctor tried putting himself in her place. He suddenly realised that during and after the war she must have seen starvation. Empathically he asked her about her war experiences and she began to soften as she spoke of people who had starved, fallen ill and gone under while she had survived.

The doctor turned to the girl who was no longer curled up like a baby in the chair but was sitting up, listening intently. 'You see what your mother has been through. You and I have never known real hunger as she has. You can see why she sometimes get so worried about eating and you must try to forgive her because you can see how difficult it must be for her to forget all she has been through.' By now mother and daughter were smiling at one another in a way the doctor had never seen before. The mother, who had come in with an inexorable demand for further referral, went out hand in hand with her daughter, all such thoughts forgotten, thanking the doctor very sincerely.

Too much must not be claimed for one brief interview, but clearly the doctor for the first time had acted therapeutically in a relationship between mother and daughter which had become progressively more disordered as the years had gone by. Instead of permitting a repetition of their fixed attitudes, he had taken the opportunity of letting mother and child see sides of each other more appropriate to their present unhappiness.

It is important to note that the interpretation was useful only as a means of altering the relationship; its content was irrelevant. In any disordered relationship it will be found that a particular situation evokes a set of attitudes in each family member towards each other member, and no one seems able to change. One aspect of the personality is conditioned always to be in charge in that situation, and it is this which the general practitioner, with his limited time but unrivalled position of authority, can help to change; only a clear demonstration of a caring and involved attitude on the part of the doctor will enable a different aspect to appear.

Joint interviews

Joint interviews are usually avoided by doctors except when the second person is needed to provide additional information. Their instinctive reaction is to deal with patients one at a time, perhaps to avoid a situation in which they are merely a third party in a squabble. There is no doubt that conducting a joint interview requires experience to obtain the best results, but many general practitioner neglect this most powerful therapeutic tool which is at their disposal.

Mr and Mrs Ormond came to talk to the doctor about their 9-year-old elder child. They drew a frightening picture of a boy with an uncontrollable temper who delighted in provoking his parents beyond endurance. The mother said, 'I have always maintained that there are no bad children, only bad parents, but we are desperate and we cannot see where we have gone wrong. We have always done our best to be kind and understanding, but he goes on and on provoking us until we lose our tempers.' The father added, 'I even tell him that if he does not mend his ways we will have to send him away, but it doesn't make any difference.' The doctor asked how long this situation had existed. 'Well, ever since he was born, really. He was a very big baby, over nine pounds, and cried a lot even in hospital; the Sister said to me, "You will never be able to manage him." It has continued like that ever since but has got worse lately. I begin to think it must be inborn. The strange thing is that we get good reports of him from school. Is that what a split personality means?'

A picture emerged of immature, insecure parents, fearful from the start of their ability to bring up a child, and of a child to whom his parents' inability to adopt an authoritative role had communicated itself as a fear that his own impulses were uncontrollable.

The doctor asked the parents to bring the boy with them the following week and the scene that ensured confirmed his impressions. After the briefest of preliminaries all three entered into an argument between themselves, virtually ignoring the doctor and brushing aside his occasional interjections. The striking feature was that the argument appeared to be between three children as equals: the boy mildly aggressive to conceal an obvious anxiety, the parents faintly reproachful but without any hint of authority. The doctor eventually asserted himself gently but firmly. Having given a demonstration of a benevolent but authoritative parent, he handed authority back to the mother and father by suggesting that the boy would find it easier if he had rules for situations that were usually difficult, transgression of which would be followed by specified punishments without argument. The doctor discussed these rules with the mother and father as parent to parent, then turned to the boy and discussed with him the difficulties of keeping a rein on his temper and other aspects of his delinquent behaviour, evoking for all three the image of a fundamentally good boy learning how to cope with his problems. When they next met both the boy and his parents seemed much happier, and a great reduction in family tension was reported.

The general practitioner, with his special position of trust and access to the family circle, is in a unique position to be able to make the diagnosis of disordered relationships within a family. Where the diagnosis is of an abnormal pattern, continued over a period of years, from which the members cannot escape without quitting the family, the doctor may be able to trigger a change in family assumptions and roles which will have profound effect on the health of all the members.

Incidental crises
Disordered relationships in a family often arise from the normal crises through which its members pass, like pregnancy, puberty,

menopause and death. Incidental and accidental crises which occur in one member of the family may present as illness in another.

> Mrs Pitt, aged 19, had married her 20-year-old husband because she was pregnant. During the pregnancy she was found to have chronic pyelonephritis. Her urine was made sterile and she was to be investigated by the hospital after her confinement.
> Eight months after delivery she complained of vague abdominal pains. When the doctor asked if she was troubled by anything she said that everything was fine.
> He commented that she still had the urinary investigations hanging over her head, and that in such circumstance he would be nervous. 'Oh, I'm not upset about that. I suppose I had better tell you. My husband has been charged with indecent exposure and has seen a psychiatrist for a court medical report. He'll be writing to you anyway.'

Mrs Pitt presented because of something which had happened to her husband; even though she knew a letter would reach the doctor she found difficulty in telling him of the occurrence. Both she and the psychiatrist attributed Mr Pitt's behaviour to an emotional crisis precipitated by learning that his wife had an unsuspected illness which had made the unintended pregnancy dangerous. Each partner showed the effects of the other's illness.

Couvade
Couvade, or sympathetic pregnancy pains, has long been recognised, although its existence is not accepted by everyone.

> Mr Quale, a skilled worker of 35, complained of dyspepsia. The history indicated duodenal ulceration and this was confirmed radiologically. His symptoms failed to respond to medical treatment, although radiologically his ulcer did. His wife was then three months pregnant. As her mild nausea of pregnancy subsided so did Mr Quale's dyspeptic symptoms, only to be replaced a few months later by palpitation and pain in the chest for which no physical cause could be found. They disappeared when the baby was born. His wife remained undisturbed by her pregnancy, but, throughout, was worried by her husband's condition.

The family size and complexity
Most of the stories we quote in this chapter relate to nuclear families and it is easy to assume that if only extended families still existed in our society, the problems of the general practitioner would be fewer. One suspects that the opposite may be true. The number of possible bonds in a family increases polynomially with the number of its members but more bonds do not necessarily mean better relationships. Every clan has a power structure—a ruler, a group of advisors, and a subject population. The roles may change for different tasks. Most doctors become familiar with an extended

family only gradually; they slowly discover the power structure within which its members function and which constrains both their assumptions and their actions.

The doctor was called late one evening to Daisy Roe, pregnant with her second child and booked for home confinement. She had been vomiting but not to a degree that justified a call. Her husband, Basil, did most of the talking and then Daisy asked for a tonic for him. The doctor asked Basil to come to the surgery. Basil came and complained of a recurrence of abdominal pain for which no cause had been found when it had been investigated a year previously. He was clinically depressed, but the doctor could establish no communication with him.

This seemed a simple case of couvade, but there were two features which disturbed the doctor: his inability to get Basil to talk, which suggested that the depression was severe, and his knowledge of Basil's parents, the Roes, and their other children.

Coral was the youngest Roe, ten years junior to Basil, and was 'always ill'. The doctors had to make frequent late visits but never really got her better. 'Your medicine didn't help her, doctor, so I stopped it and gave her . . . and now she is better, but I would like a tonic for her. The last one you gave me didn't work and I got her some . . . Could I have some of that this time?' This pattern was always repeated. The doctor eventually learnt his place. It seemed to him that being masculine in Mrs Roe's house must be depressing. She was always asking men to do things and then proving that they couldn't. This opinion had been confirmed in consultations with her husband Albert.

The doctor wondered what was happening to Basil now, since all the men in the Roe family seemed depressed anyhow. Basil did not return to the doctor. Pregnancy, however, can be a continuing crisis.

Daisy continued to visit the antenatal clinic and at one visit asked again for a tonic for her husband. The doctor tried to get her to talk about her own problem. She told him that Basil said he was upset because she was pregnant. When she had pointed out that he had agreed to have a second child, he had replied, 'Well, you wanted another one, and I thought Karen ought to have a companion.' Daisy felt that this was very unfair. The doctor repeated his suggestion that she should ask Basil to come to the surgery. He did not come.

A common ploy
This incident shows the common ploy of asking the doctor to treat an absent member of the family. Here he tried to refuse and failed.

In the event, no more was heard about the matter until Daisy was 37 weeks pregnant. The police from a neighbouring district telephoned the doctor to say that Basil had been found dead. It appeared to be a case of suicide: had the doctors prescribed any medication which might have been used? They had not.

Two days later Daisy telephoned the doctor. She said that she was upset because the police did not consult her, always ringing her brother-in-law who did not pass the messages on. She felt very excluded. The doctor pointed out that the police meant well, and asked what she felt about her in-laws. She said that they blamed her for Basil's death. The doctor gave Daisy the police telephone number, and suggested that if she contacted them they would be pleased to keep her informed and allow her to see Basil's body. Daisy said she was grateful: it was the first time in the whole business that she had felt sensible, and that made her happier. The doctor was gratified at the effect of a little common-sense advice, but then realised that Daisy herself seemed a very sensible woman. He was puzzled by her apparent need to be told what to do.

Meanwhile, the grandparents Roe were in turmoil, particularly grandmother. Her husband sent for the doctor late at night, saying she was having a breakdown. It transpired that she was crying a great deal, and playing no part in the funeral arrangements or in dealing with the police. The doctor commented that it was proper for a mother to cry when her son died, even more so perhaps if he had committed suicide. Grandmother nodded. Her husband said that she was a loving mother and that it was all Daisy's fault that Basil had committed suicide. Daisy simply had not been a proper wife to him.

Five days after Basil's suicide the doctor was consulted about his daughter Karen, aged 2, who was brought to the surgery by an elderly woman, Mrs Richards, whom the doctor guessed to be Daisy's mother. Mrs Richards said that she and Daisy were worried because Karen had woken crying the previous night and when comforted had broken into hysterical laughter. The doctor suggested that it was not surprising the child was disturbed: after all, her father had disappeared. Did she know that he was dead? It transpired that the child had first been told that her father was at work and later that he had gone away. The doctor said it appeared that Daisy was having some trouble expressing her feelings in front of the child. Mrs Richards said, 'Surely Karen isn't old enough to understand?'

Alignment or non-alignment

Mrs Richards had blithely told the doctor what they had told Karen about her father in front of the child, who was transparently able to understand what was being said. Many parents—and many doctors—make the assumption that a child cannot understand what is being said between two adults, though this is usually untrue at any age from the toddler stage onwards. A child will always detect prevarication, and, where there is deep unhappiness in the family, inevitably becomes very anxious. The doctor pointed this out to Mrs Richards, who had said that she was now living with Daisy. He was worried about the impact that the imminent birth of the new baby would have on Karen, particular if no-one was likely to explain things to her, and he did not feel able to manage the whole extended family by himself.

This is one of the predicaments of the of the general practitioner. He can usually align himself clearly on the side of his patient, but if he is dealing with a family situation it may be impossible for him to be on the same side as everyone concerned. In some cases recorded in previous chapters this was not necessary: ranging himself on one side against the other was an effective method of establishing communication. Here the doctor already had two conflicting sides to take (grandmother Roe's and Daisy's) and he did not feel capable of taking a third position.

He suggested that it might be a good idea for Mrs Richards and Daisy to obtain some help from a child psychiatrist, but was careful to add that Mrs Richards herself seemed a warm-hearted woman and would be able to show Karen the love and concern she needed in her present predicament.

'Oh yes, doctor, I love children. I'm not Karen's grandmother, I'm really her great-grandmother. Daisy's mother and father separated when her mother, my daughter, had a child by another man. Daisy and her half-sister were sent from foster home to foster home, so I adopted them, and both she and Karen call me 'Gran'.

It was agreed that Daisy would discuss the matter with the doctor a couple of days later when she was to attend his antenatal clinic. The doctor felt that he had avoided treating the absent patient while finding out a little more about Daisy's own family and bringing Mrs Richards into his picture of what was going on. At the interview with Daisy it was agreed that arrangements should be made for Karen to see a child psychiatrist. It became obvious that Daisy was indeed as intelligent and capable of being competent as the doctor thought, but she always seemed to need a man to say 'Yes, you are right,'

This was highlighted when Daisy got into an argument with her in-laws on a subject of some importance to her during a week-end when the doctor was not available. She found out from Mrs Richards the address of her true father whom she had not seen for years and who had re-married, spoke to him and obtained his approval for her stand against her in-laws.

The doctor pointed out that she knew that should be done each time, and was usually right, but there did seem to be this need to get a man to endorse her decisions before she could take action. She readily agreed that this was so. 'When my father left my mother I was 3 and when I asked why he had gone, I was told it was because my mother had done wrong. I suppose she had, but I've never realised before how this has always coloured my thinking.'

The doctor said: 'Well, that should make you realise it's important for Karen to get her father's death and the new birth straight in her mind.' 'Yes, doctor, of course I realise that. That was why I asked Gran to bring Karen to you 'But you didn't ask me outright to do something; you left it up to me.' 'Yes, but I knew you would do what you did.'

Working in tandem

At this point the doctor saw something very important. He knew that Basil had come from a family where the men were told to do things and made to feel frustrated. Daisy, on the other hand, believed that even though she knew what should be done she should never appear to be in control, and in fact would not even make a suggestion when she knew what ought to be done. This meant that the marriage of Basil and Daisy would have been one which appeared very quiet and pleasant whilst in fact each waited unhappily for the other to take the initiative and assume control. This seemed to be confirmed by Basil's statement about the conception of the expected baby.

The doctor pointed out the situation as it appeared to him. Daisy eagerly agreed. He then remarked that she now seemed to be using him as the person to take control, but that really he had been unable to manage by himself and had had to turn to the psychiatrist and to Mrs Richards and to Daisy herself. Perhaps it was not true what either she or Basil had thought, but that men and women needed to work in tandem.

Throughout Daisy's difficulties in the succeeding months the doctor, when asked, would take positive action but would always point out that Daisy had already decided and usually achieved the ends she sought. Daisy gradually became able to manage her own affairs on her own initiative.

This case shows several of the classic traps for the general practitioner. There were clear-cut power structures in the extended family on each side, one of which was known to the doctor. At the point where the families met—in the marriage of Basil and Daisy—there was bound to be trouble. In many cases the conflict is sorted out in the 'honeymoon period' but in the marriage of Basil and Daisy it never became overt and the result was tragic.

The 'absent patient'

The harm which is done to children when they are given misleading or false information about important events in their lives is well demonstrated. The initial consultation was an example of the presenting patient not always being the one who is most ill, and there were several instances of invitations to treat 'the absent patient'—situations which need to be distinguished from each other. If the doctor colludes with the patient to put the blame on a third party he may end by offering inappropriate sympathy and missing the chance to do something more useful.

Family therapy

Techniques for treating disturbed relationships in families are now well-developed (Minuchin & Fishman 1981), and some general practitioners may wish to acquire them. All general practitioners need to be aware of what goes on in families and to build up a picture of those with which he is most explicitly involved. At the moment the claim most of us make to be family doctors is ill-founded. The intermeshing of the cogs in a family is as nicely adjusted as in a fine timepiece. Few of us are skilled enough to make delicate adjustments to such complex mechanisms, but we should at least be aware of the risks we are forced to take when we shake a family by treating one member or commenting on others. Shaking will not necessarily help them keep time with each other.

Reference

Minuchin S, Fishman H C 1981 Family Therapy Techniques. Harvard University Press, London.

12

Health breaking through

A patient who complains that the scar from his recent operation is itching is likely to be told that this is a good sign: it means that healing is taking place. Whether or not the explanation is correct, it shows that we are willing to entertain the idea that a return to health can cause symptoms.

> Susan Anderson, aged 20, was attractive and well-educated and worked as a 'girl Friday' to the production manager of a small recording company. She had not consulted a doctor for seven years, but was now complaining of headaches, tight feelings in her stomach and difficulty in getting to sleep—all becoming worse in the last month or so. Having first denied that she had any worries she went on to describe a situation that was causing her considerable stress.
>
> She was living with her boyfriend, a singer in a pop group who kept very late hours and was often away from home. He expected her to look after all his needs instantly and was extremely jealous. Her employer was also exploiting her, but she put up with this because he was good at his job and she wanted to learn enough to pursue her own career. The demands of these two men on her often conflicted, leaving her tense and miserable.
>
> The doctor asked Susan why she put up with their selfish behaviour. She said she supposed she had been brought up to expect it: her father had treated her mother and herself in a similar way, and she wondered if she could ever escape the effects of this conditioning. The doctor replied that her symptoms might mean she was already rebelling against it, and that she needed encouragement rather than treatment.
>
> The idea that they were a sign of health breaking through was difficult for her at first, but the more she thought about it the more she liked it. She went out looking pleased, and the doctor never saw her again. Six months later one of her friends told the doctor that Susan had moved, taken a new job and seemed happy.

After the consultation the doctor wondered why it had been so successful. Any of Susan's girl-friends could and would have encouraged her to assert herself. Perhaps his contribution had been the idea that her distressing symptoms were due to growing up rather than cracking up, an idea for which she was ready and which gave her hope. He thought that other patients might be able to use it too. Soon afterwards he met Mrs Burns, whose problems were to involve him for more than a year.

Pamela Burns, aged 48, had been getting repeat prescriptions for sleeping tablets for ten years, usually without a consultation. One evening she came to ask the doctor, who was new to the practice, for a further supply. She resisted his attempt to discuss the request in a way he found defiant and challenging rather than agressive. Eventually he agreed to it on condition that she come back to tell him what was going on and see if it might be possible for her to give them up.

In the interviews which followed the doctor learned her story. He felt that despite her protestations she was glad to be forced to tell it.

She had made a disastrous marriage at the age of 19 to a man who turned out to be a sexual sadist, and only her naive optimism enabled the marriage to last for two years. Her sexual feelings seemed to have been normal at first, but after the divorce all that remained of them was a sense of total revulsion.

Six years later Mrs Burns married again, mainly because she was lonely. Her second husband was willing to wait until she was ready for intercourse. She was affected by his patience and consideration, and felt very guilty about the way she reacted to any physical intimacy. Over the next four years she slowly relaxed, but just when she was sure that everything was going to be all right, her husband died suddenly of a heart attack, the marriage still unconsummated. Her guilt intensified, and she determined never to have another close relationship with a man. She put her energies into her job, got some enjoyment from flirting with the men at work, started going to evening classes and went out only with women.

Some seven years later she began to find she could not get to sleep and started taking nitrazepam. Several attempts to do without the drug had been abandoned because she was too tired to work in the day-time, and after so many years she was now frightened of trying again.

The doctor still had the feeling that Mrs Burns wanted him to make her try, and he insisted that she wean herself off the nitrazepam fairly quickly. She continued to make her regular appointments, in which she talked about her current problems and always told him how hard he was in depriving her of her sleep. After six months of this she said that she could not come back to him any more because she was in love with him.

The doctor said he thought that this was an important development. It had taken ten years for her frozen feelings to thaw out after her divorce, and when they had become too strong for her to cope with she had started to take nitrazepam. Without the sleeping tablets they were active again, and he was a safe recipient for them because she knew that nothing would happen as a result. It seemed to him that health was breaking through irresistibly and he was happy for her to continue her visits for as long as she found them helpful.

Mrs Burns did keep coming back, though gradually less often. After six months she told the doctor that she had met someone very special and was going to be married very soon. Sex has not presented any problems in her third marriage, and she has since said that she recognised the truth of the idea of health breaking through as soon as it was put to her, though nothing would have induced her to admit it then. This, and the doctor's willingness to carry on because he believed in it, had made her feel safe and had given her strength while the final stages of battles against her resistance to becoming normal again were taking place.

It seems that the concept of 'health breaking through' is useful to someone who is making a painful transition from a long-standing unhealthy emotional state to a more normal one. It offers more than the simple explanation that the symptoms being experienced are a reaction to stress, because it puts them into a perspective that is both dynamic and hopeful.

It is unlikely to help patients who are not already in transit: for example those who ask for treatment because they want to go on playing the martyr in more comfort. Susan Anderson and Pamela Burns would almost certainly have recovered without the doctor's intervention; he jumped on a rolling bandwagon and perhaps moved it along a little faster. He also prevented their problems from being defined in medical terms and treated with drugs.

There is another rather different syndrome with which 'health breaking through' should not be confused. In this the patient goes on experiencing symptoms after their cause has been cured—they have become no more than an unnecessary habit. This is a static situation, unlike the dynamic process of 'health breaking through', and when diagnosed accurately responds quickly to the doctor's 'permission to get better', much to everyone's surprise.

EMOTIONAL MATURITY

The story of Susan Anderson in particular raises the question of what we mean by the term 'emotional maturity'. It is really no more than a concept invented to explain some of the behaviour we observe, but it is useful because of the order it allows us to impose. We can see circumstances as a stimulus, behaviour as a response, and emotions as an intervening variable—and a lack of events or an inability to do anything about one's circumstances may constitute a situation just as stressful as any dramatic happening. With this simple sequence we can define some of the terms found in other chapters of this book and elsewhere in medical writing.

Anxiety is what we feel when we wonder how we will cope with a new experience we see looming ahead. Whether we are feeling anxiety, boredom or frustration, *neurotic behaviour* consists of responding to circumstances in set ways which are inappropriate. *'Health breaking through'* occurs as we dimly recognise that we have become able to cope with our circumstances and have no further use for our neurotic behaviour.

Discovering that we can cope gets rid of our anxiety, and in one area of our personality at least we become more mature. *Emotional insecurity* means that we are struggling to function at a level of maturity which we have not attained in enough areas.

When we fail to cope we *regress*, and this presents several possibilities. Regressing may make us more secure, so that we are not interested in struggling to cope—other people are then likely to say that we have an *indequate personality*, though this will provoke anxiety only if we are not really more comfortable at the lower level of functioning. Alternatively we may obtain social approval for regressing if we are designated as *ill*, though the illness must not go on for longer than other people think proper. Either way, our self-esteem is not damaged and the experience has brought us some gain.

If we regard the experience as a loss, the scene is set for *depression*. If the loss seems to be due to external circumstances we tend to complain and exhibit *helplessness*; if we blame ourselves we feel guilty and worthless, and because no-one can put things right we feel *hopeless* or even suicidal. Furthermore, since loss is quite a frequent occurrence, and if we are poor at adapting, we are liable to suffer from *recurrent depression*.

When we get old we try to arrange life so that we have as few new experiences as possible, because this makes it easier to maintain our existing equilibrium. This arrangement is discussed in Chapter 15 as *social disengagement*.

13

Anxiety

People feel anxious when events or changes in their lives disturb their emotional equilibrium. The extent to which an individual can meet his anxiety with constructive action defines the level of his emotional maturity, and he becomes emotionally more mature when he copes successfully with a situation that is making him anxious.

In this sense the situation itself is neutral—it is the individual's reaction to which we attach significance and apply judgement, and the English language is rich in phrases which recognise this. Being got out of one's rut, knocked off one's pedestal, caught on the hop, bowled over or given a push (whether forward or over the edge) may all be destabilising experiences, but each carries a different implication. The anxiety attending them is therefore something to be assessed: if symptoms are invariably treated with anxiolytic drugs, many patients will be denied the chance of achieving equilibrium at a more mature level, and some may regress to a less mature level because their drive to cope with a new situation has been taken away.

Mrs Allen, aged 38, was a new patient who had left her husband and family near Swindon and had been living with her lover in London for 18 months. She told the doctor that she had been anxious before she made the move and that she had been prescribed a benzodiazepine by her previous doctor. Her two daughters, aged 15 and 13, wanted to live with her rather than with their father, since he had brought into the house a 20-year-old girl whom he intended to marry when his divorce came through. Mrs Allen's lover apparently had no intention of marrying her, although their relationship was settling down.

Mrs Allen said that she had been very reluctant to threaten her burgeoning relationship with new responsibilities and had taken some of the tranquillisers that remained from her previous treatment. Perhaps as a consequence, she had dallied and dithered, giving no answer to her daughters, making no mention to her lover of her daughters' wishes, and effectively ignoring a letter from her husband's lawyer concerning the custody of the children. With only two days to go before she had to appear in court, she was asking the doctor what he thought she ought to do. It seemed to him that if she had not taken the tranquillisers she might have shown some concern a little earlier.

Anxiety is most often presented to the general practitioner by patients who are faced with the need to make decisions.

Mrs Bell, aged 31, was brought to the surgery by a neighbour who said that she had had a 'fit'. Mrs Bell was weeping brokenly, and told her story in little bursts. She was five days overdue and she couldn't possibly have another baby: she couldn't stand the thought of it. On the other hand, if she turned out to be pregnant she couldn't stand the thought of a termination either. She had tried to commit suicide two nights earlier but the aspirins had made her sick before she could take enough of them.

Mrs Bell was faced with what seemed to her to be two totally unacceptable alternatives. Her anxiety was so overwhelming that she had made a serious attempt on her own life: a logical solution perhaps when a symptom seems unbearable and incurable. Her response serves as an illustration of the Yerkes-Dodson law which states that increasing arousal at first improves performance but later leads to a deterioration as emotion disrupts behaviour. The more complex the task, the lower is the optimal level of arousal for effective performance.

Mrs Allen and Mrs Bell were strangers to the doctor when they presented with their crises. Had he known them longer he might have developed a feel for the sort of situations with which they could not cope, and by anticipatory discussion prevented their situations from appearing as crises at all.

Handicapping or helpful

Deciding whether anxiety is helpful or handicapping is a major task for any general practitioner. What guidelines can he use? Relying on generalisations such as 'most patients aren't as anxious as this about this sort of thing' does not take him very far. Since the degree of anxiety which a patient feels and the level to which it is tolerable are both related to the personality and previous experience of the individual as well as to the provoking event, this kind of generalisation is unhelpful; nor does it explain the form that the anxiety takes, which may be anything from a severe monosymptomatic phobia to a mild generalised anxiety. It certainly does not suggest what method of management is likely to the most appropriate. Different theories of anxiety offer different ways of understanding it, and three of these ways may be of particular service to the doctor both in deciding whether a particular patient's anxiety is handicapping or helpful, and in making decisions about its management.

Conflict and anxiety

Human beings can be considered as goal-directed, in that they seek either to approach or to avoid particular ends. At the most basic level, a person may be motivated to search for food to assuage hunger or shelter to avoid cold and damp, but in our society motivations are usually much more complex than this. Conflict arises if someone is motivated simultaneously towards two incompatible goals (approach–approach conflict), if he is driven simultaneously both to do and not to do something (approach–avoidance conflict) or if he is faced by a situation the resolutions to which are all to some extent unacceptable (avoidance–avoidance conflict).

When anxiety appears to be the result of one of these kinds of conflict, the logical way of dealing with it is to reach a decision about the best available compromise between the warring aims. When the patient can understand all the factors that have to be taken into account, he needs counselling—a highly skilled but psychologically superficial process which makes him evaluate thoroughly for himself the relative importance of each of the factors. If, as is often the case, he has mysterious emotional blocks that prevent him from accepting a compromise or solution which he can see intellectually to be appropriate, it is likely that he needs some kind of interpretive psychotherapy. Anxiolytic drugs have a place only for a brief period while he is being brought back into that critical part of the Yerkes-Dodson curve where he has enough arousal to learn—not so much that it gets in the way, and not so little that his motivation to learn is flattened.

Approach–approach conflict

Miss Cullen, aged 21, had two young children and no regular relationship with a partner. She consulted the doctor because she had symptoms which sounded as though they were due to anxiety. She said that she was worried because she did not know what to do. She had at last been offered the new Council accommodation for which she had been pressing for some time. The date on which she was supposed to move came in the middle of the first holiday she had been able to arrange since the birth of her first child three years earlier. There were no factors in either choice which seemed unacceptable to her: she simply saw the two goals, new accommodation and a holiday, as incompatible, though she very much wanted both. Her degree of anxiety was not high; nor, in the event, were the two goals really incompatible.

Miss Cullen seems to have been faced with an approach–approach conflict. Despite many other anxiety-provoking features in her life she did not appear unduly anxious, although she *did* appear crippled in her decision-making. It is a reasonably sound general rule that if a patient presents an approach–approach conflict as the cause of overt anxiety then either the true conflict has not been identified or the patient has a generalised anxiety trait.

Approach–avoidance conflict

Mr Doyle, aged 50, had suffered from low-backache for years. The doctor had the impression that the backache appeared whenever Mr Doyle was given a little more responsibility than usual for his job as a fitter in a garage. He was a conscientious worker—a little obsessive in fact; perhaps this limited the amount of responsibility he could tolerate. In the fullness of time Mr Doyle was offered promotion to foreman. 'The work is lighter, it will be good for your back and of course you will earn more money,' he reported his employer as saying.

Mr Doyle presented to the doctor in acute anxiety. He wanted to keep his job and not be promoted. How was he to refuse promotion without losing his job, especially in view of what his employer had said about his back?

This is a classic approach–avoidance conflict. Of course categorising it in this way does not account for every question that arises—the origin of Mr Doyle's tendency towards obsession and where he learnt to use his back as an instrument for playing the sick role, for example; what the categorisation does is to direct attention towards the kind of management most likely to be helpful. The doctor might have been able to guess that such a situation was bound to occur eventually for a man like Mr Doyle.

Avoidance–avoidance conflict

Avoidance-avoidance conflict is illustrated by Mrs Bell who faced alternatives (abortion or another child) which were both unacceptable to her. The anxiety aroused by avoidance–avoidance conflicts is often very intense, as it was for her, but resolution is almost inevitable if the anxiety can be supported in the meantime.

Multiple conflicts

All doctors will recognise that many patients experience approach–avoidance conflicts of a multiple nature. This is hardly surprising in view of the complex nature of our society and the wide range of demands it makes upon individuals.

Mrs Earle, a 62-year-old widow, consulted the doctor in a state of marked anxiety and with all the usual symptoms. 'I know you'll think I'm silly. You know I lost my husband when Jacqui, the youngest of my three daughters, was only 2 years old. You know Jacqui has a 6-month-old baby, Mark. I babysat for them three months ago—he's a lovely boy. All the time I was waiting for Jacqui and her husband to come home I was worried about Mark. He was breathing funny but I didn't want to interfere. I've always tended to make a baby out of Jacqui and now she's married I try not to interfere: she's got to grow up and lead her own life, especially now she's a mother herself. I'd *offered* to babysit; it was the first time they had been out together since Mark was born and that wasn't right so I *had* pressed them a bit. Anyhow when Jacqui came home I told her I was worried about Mark and that they should call their doctor. Mark was rushed to hospital with bronchitis and was very ill. I knew I should have done something myself but I didn't want to interfere. Jacqui doesn't blame me at all. In fact she keeps asking me to babysit again but I'm too frightened to, and now they can't go out at all and they're beginning to squabble. I'm frightened their marriage will break up, and I don't know what to do!'

The series of approach–avoidance conflicts is self-evident. Mrs Earle's anxieties also suggest a second way of considering anxiety: that related to the concept of defence mechanisms.

Defence mechanisms

Defences are an integral part of the structure of every personality: their existence is not of necessity pathological. A defence mechanism is a manoeuvre by which the expression is prevented of an impulse or wish which is unacceptable to an individual for a variety of personal reasons. We are not usually conscious of our defence mechanisms and if they are called into question we tend to feel anxious without knowing quite why. It is socially unacceptable to be anxious without a reason, so if our unconscious defence mechanisms begin to let us down we first try to conceal our anxiety. If we cannot hide it we may try to rationalise it by attaching it to something which we do know we are concerned about or we may go further and displace it on to some external object or situation which we then avoid—a phobia.

The concept of defence mechanisms stems from psychoanalytical theory, as does the idea of displacement as the cause of phobias. Anxiety which has no clear focus can sometimes be understood and helped by forms of psychotherapy far briefer than psychoanalysis, in terms of the failure of habitual defence mechanisms like repression, denial, rationalisation, projection, regression, reaction formation, introjection and sublimation. Phobias, on the other hand, seemed to be managed best by some kind of desensitisation technique based on learning theory.

Mrs France, aged 28, registered with the doctor and consulted him at the same visit. She asked for a combined analgesic tablet which she took regularly and described the classical physical symptoms of anxiety: dizziness, palpitations, difficulty in breathing, sweating, going hot and cold, and so on. Her manner was eager but diffident. The general practitioner asked Mrs France to explain why she needed the tablets. She told him that she suffered from a rare genetic disease which had left her partly-sighted since birth. When she was 6 years old she had been knocked down by a lorry, and her right leg had been saved from amputation by a series of operations over the next 20 years. Under her trousers her right leg was grossly deformed and the doctor happily gave her the analgesic. She then went on to talk about being brought up by her blind parents with her two partly-sighted sisters. The doctor noted that Mrs France displayed very little emotion while she was telling her story. The doctor did not understand the reasons for Mrs France's presenting symptoms of anxiety and asked why she had moved to his practice area. 'Oh,' she said, still with no emotion, 'my husband beat me up so often that he was put in prison. My social worker thought I ought to move so that when he came out he wouldn't find me easily. He's out of prison now. I've had to change my job too.'

The doctor suggested that her symptoms of palpitations, dizziness, and so on might be associated with all the difficulties she had described. Mrs France looked at him blankly: 'I don't understand what you mean doctor,' and went on to talk briskly about the pain in her leg and the pleasure she got from her new job as a care assistant for elderly people.

Over the next 12 months Mrs France reduced her need for analgesics but still consulted quite frequently. Each consultation followed the same pattern: she would first present a new and 'real' physical problem like a left carpal tunnel syndrome, low-backache with left sciatica and limited straight raising of the left leg, and giant urticaria. On each occasion she would mention episodes of dizziness and palpitations for which the doctor find no organic cause, and on each occasion she would, without any obvious emotion, describe situations involving her husband, her sight, her right leg, and her new job which most people would have found anxiety-provoking. On each occasion she would look blankly at the doctor if he suggested there might be an association between some of her symptoms and the situation(s) in which she found herself.

It appeared that Mrs France was able successfully to repress for quite long periods the anxieties and self-doubts which would have beset most people in her situation. It seemed probable that she had acquired skills in this particular defence mechanism during a life time of unfortunate happenings and frightening operations. The doctor continued to care for Mrs France on the basis of each new 'real' complaint, never pushing very hard for the source of the continuing symptoms which he was sure were due to anxiety. He wondered how long she would be able to use her preferred defence successfully and noted when her records reached him that as a teenager she had twice had hospital admissions for a depressive illness.

Mrs France's doctor is waiting to see if her defences will one day prove insufficient and if she will become depressed again.

Learning theory

Learning theory may be encapsulated in the proposition that behaviour is governed by its consequences. The theory is based mainly on the concept of operant conditioning, which in turn is based on the idea of classifying the consequences of behaviour as: positively reinforcing (gaining pleasure or reward); negatively reinforcing (getting rid of discomfort or unpleasantness); or punishing (experiencing discomfort as a result of persisting in a behaviour). These three possible types of outcome can be used both to explain the development of some behaviours and also to ablate them.

> Miss George, aged 31, registered with the doctor and consulted him about symptoms which were due to acute cholecystitis. She lived by herself with no friends or relations nearby. The doctor recorded in his notes that she had not once looked him in the eye.
> He saw Miss George again after her discharge from hospital; this time she confided in him that she became extremely anxious when she entered an underground train or a large and crowded supermarket. She had found her experiences in tube trains so uncomfortable that she avoided them and had switched to the bus, even though it took her an hour longer to get to and from work. Then she began to experience the same symptoms in crowded buses, and left her highly-paid job in the City for a local post with much lower pay. Her problems in adjusting to her lower income were compounded by her inability to shop in supermarkets, which forced her to rely on more expensive 'corner shops'. Her salary had not been paid whilst she was in hospital and the consequent financial short-fall seemed to have forced her into presenting the problem to the doctor.

The concept of reinforcement (positive and negative) describes rather than explains the relationship between two classes of events (Winefield & Peay 1980). Nevertheless, it allows for some prediction and control of the behaviour involved. In terms of learning theory it can be suggested that whatever the trigger for Miss George's fear of crowded places, she had negatively reinforced the tendency by repeatedly exposing herself to the unpleasant feeling aroused by entering tubes, buses and supermarkets and then giving herself relief by removing herself from the situation. The treatment which follows logically from this idea is to desensitise the patient by avoiding the negative reinforcement, making her stay longer in the unpleasant situation. This requires a careful gradation of the situations in terms of their unpleasantness. It may be too much to expect someone to tolerate the extra unpleasantnesses involved without there being anyone with her to hold her hand, literally as well as metaphorically. If the patient has a strong dependent relationship with the doctor, desensitisation can be used without the doctor physically accompanying the patient into the anxiety-provoking situations. Fortunately phobic people seem easily able to form dependent relationships and the rewards to both patient and doctor of desensitisation are so high that the activity can soon become positively reinforcing for both.

> The doctor and Miss George made a detailed behavioural analysis of the situations which produced her anxiety. They selected for the mode of

desensitisation her fear of supermarkets, partly because a large modern shopping centre lay a quarter of a mile from the practice premises. The agreement was that she would see him in the surgery, be given a task of selected difficulty (going to the centre for instance, and looking into a supermarket, for five minutes) and then returning to receive his congratulations. Within two months of short sessions, during ordinary consulting hours, Miss George's major symptoms were under control.

It is obvious that Miss George's problem can also be described in terms of defence mechanisms: an unacceptable wish or impulse being first *repressed* and then, as this mechanism failed, being *displaced* on to an external situation which in turn set the scene for *avoidance*. It is often difficult to base rapid effective treatment of disabling phobias on explanations concerning defence mechanism. Equally well, treatment of a phobia by behavioural methods ignores the unacceptable wish which is believed to be its real cause, so that there may be a need for the feelings involved to be discussed as well. The 'how' of behavioural therapy does not necessarily exclude the 'why' of psycho-analytical theory; 'how' therapy can so strengthen the doctor-patient relationship that the no longer overtly disabled patient becomes able to uncover the repressed 'why' of his or her phobic condition.

In practice, few general practitioners are so wedded to any rigid school of thought that they feel bound to interpret the problems of each anxious patient in terms of conflict, defence mechanisms, learning theory or any other abstract concept. As patients' stories emerge, the most appropriate model tends to suggest itself quite naturally, and often the doctor will recognise what form of management is indicated without realising that he has understood the situation in the terms of whichever model logically goes with such management.

Nor are these models always helpful: there are times when none of them seems to fit the case, when there is no ascertainable answer to 'why?' and no clear pattern to 'when?' the symptoms occur. The doctor may be forced to conclude that he is dealing with someone who has an anxious personality and that there is no point in searching for any specific focus. In psychological parlance, anxiety can be a 'trait' as well as a 'state'.

Mr Haynes, aged 34, was brought to the surgery by his wife. 'He's always tired and he snaps at me. He doesn't seem to care for me any more. He's always walking around the house and can't sit still. He never finishes anything he starts. He gets these palpitations at night and there's times when he can't breathe. He thinks he's going to die when he gets these attacks.'
Mr Haynes was a little man; his wife was a big woman. He had been sitting, careworn, wringing his hands, wriggling in his chair and looking back

and forth between the doctor and his wife. 'Yes,' he chimed in, 'I really feel like I'm going to die. It's like I'm always worried, but I've got nothing to worry about, really. It's always been a bit like this; it's getting worse since we had to move back in with my wife's mother when my father-in-law died.'

Mr Haynes's wriggling and other behaviour seemed childlike. Certainly it could be postulated that the gap between the maturity he was required to evince and the maturity he actually felt was so great that he was perpetually insecure and anxious, but this hypothesis would not help much in his management. Discussing the exacerbation of his symptoms which took place when he went to live with his mother-in-law might bring a little relief, but few doctors would expect it to 'cure' him.

It may be more useful to see Mr Haynes as having an autonomic nervous system which was both over-sensitive to triggers and highly reactive, so that his symptoms became self-reinforcing: the thought of experiencing the physical symptoms of anxiety would make him anxious.

Mild generalised anxiety is sometimes treated on this basis with benzodiazepines to reduce the symptoms experienced; unfortunately, patients frequently become habituated to benzodiazepine, with the result that they experience symptoms like those for which they were originally treated as soon as the drug is withdrawn, a confusing situation which usually lasts for about a month. If the withdrawal response does not disappear spontaneously, the doctor has one of two choices: to prescribe the tranquilliser again, for the use only when the symptoms are unbearable, or to find a totally different approach.

Thoughts which accompany the feelings of anxiety seem to be easily forgotten by people who have a mild anxiety trait, and it is this phenomenon which makes rational discussion with the patient about his condition so difficult. Studies of the way people remember seem to suggest that there is a stage at which items for recall are stored in 'the brain' in a private language (often called a metalanguage). If the thought or topic associated with the feelings of anxiety has a private language label which has not been translated into English, the patient will not be able to tell anyone else what it is.

Beck & Emery (1979) suggested a new approach to anxiety and phobic disorders which they called 'cognitive therapy'. Matthews (1982) describes the underlying assumptions of this therapy as being that 'processes such as stereotyped thoughts, irrational beliefs and interpretive biases either control or modify anxiety'. The therapeutic approach is basically educational and is of stipulated duration involving 10–15 interviews and based on a collaborative relationship between doctor and patient. Treatment always involves the same sequence of steps. The patient must be helped to identify any thoughts related in time to the experience of anxiety. This can often be achieved by asking the patient to keep a diary in which he records any thoughts he can immediately he is aware of an exacerbation of his anxiety. At the next interview the patient discusses these thoughts with the doctor. The doctor attempts to have the patient reveal any intellectual associations between thought and worry. The patient is then encouraged to question the validity of any assumptions or beliefs which are revealed by these associations and the doctor offers alternatives to the patient to help the development of more profitable beliefs. These are reinforced by the patient doing 'homework' set by the doctor. Cognitive therapy seems to have an intellectual connection to Berne's Structural Analysis: the doctor attempts to mobilise the patient's Adult to use it to identify the adverse instructions of the Parent or Child with the intention of rectifying the balance.

Coda

Many theories have been put forward to 'explain' anxiety and the behaviour that accompanies it, and it is not always necessary to understand them in making use of the treatments which are based upon them. The pragmatic doctor may take heart from the message enshrined in Festinger's Theory of Cognitive Dissonance (1957): it states that people become biassed in favour of conclusions they have already reached, or in other words, they tend to become less anxious when they reach a decision about what they are going to do, regardless of how suitable the decision may be.

References

Winefield H R, Peay M Y 1980 Behavioural science in medicine. George Allen and Unwin, London, p 79
Beck A T, Emery G 1979 Cognitive therapy of anxiety and phobic disorders. Centre for Cognitive Therapy, Philadelphia
Matthews A 1982 Cognitive therapy for general anxiety. Privately circulated
Festinger L 1957 A theory of cognitive dissonance. Row, Peterson, Evanston, Illinois

14

Children

A general practitioner is most effective when his patients co-operate with him actively, but a unique combination of circumstances makes it hard to attain this kind of relationship with children. First, it is always someone else—an 'intermediary'—who defines them as ill and presents them to the doctor; secondly they are at a stage in their lives when rapid changes are taking place, and these can be misinterpreted as 'illness'; and thirdly, his own services are bypassed by many of the other services which exist in the community.

The intermediary

Intermediaries are usually the people who have defined the child as ill. The less that the doctor agrees with the definition, the more likely he is to think that it is the intermediary who needs attention. Often one of his chief priorities is to decide who is the patient: attention can be focussed on the child, on the person who has defined the child as ill, or on the family unit as a whole. Which he chooses depends not only on the circumstances of the case and on the way he prefers to work, but also upon the kind of relationship he establishes with the child. By talking only to the intermediary, over the child's head, he rules out the possibility of getting the child's active co-operation, and this effectively reduces his options.

In the following story, the doctor chose to take the child as the patient, though it was clear that the 'illness' was an expression of parental problems.

Mrs Astley, a 37-year-old divorcee presented her son John, aged 7½, because he had abdominal pain. The complaint, present on and off, had been offered to the practice four times in two years, but not to this doctor. A careful history convinced the doctor that the symptoms did not indicate significant organic disorder. On examination he found a small right inguinal hernia which had previously gone unnoticed, but this did not seem to be related to the pain and he thought it safe to defer surgical treatment. After some discussion an agreement was reached with John and his mother: she would keep a diary of events and pains; he would make some drawings and bring them to the doctor. At this point Mrs Astley asked John to wait outside the consulting room. She told the doctor that John tended to get his pains before his father came to take him out, by arrangement, on occasional weekends. The pains also occurred when she had rows over the telephone with his father, as she sometimes did when maintenance was not paid. Mrs Astley said she still loved her husband, but he was a liar and drunkard who was always getting them into debt and she had had no choice but to divorce him. He often let John down after promising to take him out at a weekend.

John came to see the doctor three times in all, bringing drawings which which were unusual for a child of his age. The stories he told the doctor about the drawings were remarkably imaginative, very detailed, and rattled off almost without pause to draw breath. He seemed to be regurgitating something he had memorised. All the stories had a theme in common. They concerned good children, bad children and loss. Loss was sometimes by death and sometimes by cruelty, but no story made a connection between loss and punishment: good children and bad children both lost out. The doctor commented on the first occasion that the figures in the drawings had no arms: John said simply that he had forgotten to draw them—and continued to forget. On the second occasion the doctor commented on the lack of connection between 'good', 'bad' and 'losses' and John said 'Yes . . . Can I tell you my next story please?' The third time, John told two more stories which were a little less sad and then said to the doctor 'I'm not going to have any more tummyaches. I don't think I'll come back.' The hernia was dealt with some months later.

The doctor had no idea what had been going on in John's mind, but the changes that took place in him seemed to have been assisted by the decision to take him as the patient.

Rapid changes and sensitive periods

An individual's physical, psychological and social states are like systems which are in constant motion, and each affects the others. They alter at different rates in different phases of his life-cycle. When there is a phase of rapid change he is more likely to be sensitive to disturbances than when change is more gradual. In children, rapid change in more than one system is likely to be taking place. This poses problems for the doctor in at least two ways, First it is possible for parent or doctor to confuse normal development with pathological change; secondly, either doctor or parent may assume, incorrectly, that a major change in a young child must have a major cause. Either difficulty may make a doctor intervene unneccessarily or even unhelpfully.

Mrs Ball, a 28-year-old social worker, presented her feverish 5-year-old daughter Gillian. She said in passing that Gillian had begun wetting the bed again since she had started school full-time a few days earlier and that she had come home with wet pants the previous day. Mrs Ball had attributed this loss of control to the child's social changes and had decided to ignore it. Now that Gillian was feverish she was less sure.

The doctor was faced with the same problem as the mother. He felt he had no choice but to arrange for urine tests, take decisions as to treatment and advise Mrs Ball to keep her daughter away from school whatever the effect upon her social adjustment.

Services that bypass the general practitioner

In theory at least, an advantage of the British system of providing medical care by a two-tier system of primary generalists and secondary specialists is that the generalist acts as a communication centre and is able to ensure that all the information available about a patient is utilised. When the general practitioner is bypassed, a child may be put unnecessarily at risk, or the parents may be given unnecessary anxiety.

> The general practitioner made a routine postnatal visit to Mrs Camberley and her 7-day-old son Tom as soon as they were discharged from hospital. After examining the baby the doctor made a note that both testes were in the scrotum. He was chagrined to be consulted a year later by a very anxious Mrs Camberley when a Clinical Medical Officer who had been unable to bring Tom's left testis down into the scrotum referred him to a surgeon.

Three questions

In a consultation with a patient of any age a general practitioner does well to have three questions in the back of his mind: Why bring this problem? Why bring this problem to me? Why bring this problem today? The constraints imposed on consultations with children by the intermediary, the sensitive phases and the bypass mechanisms extend and complicate the range of answers to these questions.

> Colin Dilley, aged 9, was brought by his mother to the doctor, who had met neither of them before. Colin wriggled in his chair, face, limbs and body in constant movement; his mother sat still, stony-faced but despairing. 'Colin can't sit still,' began Mrs Dilley, and it was certainly true at that moment. To the doctor the movements did not seem like athetosis, chorea or any kind of tic or spasm. As soon as he turned to Colin and asked if he was, really, unable to keep still, Colin stopped wriggling, leaned forward and began to speak in a great rush but quite coherently. This was in great contrast to Mrs Dilley's slow and measured (?depressed) delivery as she went on to tell the doctor that Colin had been wriggling like this for some months. No it wasn't any worse. He had always been a nervous, restless and difficult child, very different from his placid 7-year-old only sib, Helen.

The doctor could not help wondering 'Why today?' If behaviour *is* communication, and the purposes of communication are to convey information and to make the other person act and feel in certain ways, what was the purpose of Colin's wriggling?

He asked what had led them to consult 'today', taking care to address his question to the gap between Colin and his mother. They told him that Colin had been booked to go on a school outing, had misbehaved just before it took place and had then lied about his misbehaviour. When the teacher had caught Colin out in his lie, he had been reported to the head teacher with a request that he should not be allowed to go on the outing.

The doctor wondered why he had been chosen to deal with the problem, if indeed he had been.

'What would you like me to do,' he asked, again aiming his question at the gap between Colin and his mother. What it boiled down to, according to Colin, was that the doctor should tell his teacher that he hadn't meant to lie, but had misunderstood the teacher's question. The teacher was new to Colin, very different from his previous teacher. 'Much more strict,' commented Mrs Dilley.

The doctor decided to focus on Colin's problem with his teacher, since what he had learned so far was scarcely his business.

Colin explained that he had not done some homework because he did not know how to, even though the method had been covered in class. Then he had lied about why he did not have the work ready to hand in. The doctor said that it seemed a silly thing to have done since he was bound to be found out. 'Oh', said Mrs Dilley, 'he lies all the time! He keeps stealing things as well.'

The doctor began to wish that he had not sought answers to his threee questions. They seemed to be a long way from defining the problem sufficiently, let alone finding a solution or implementing it. He should not have been surprised to elicit the last, apparently disastrous, piece of information. Mrs Dilley had pointed out early in the consultation that Colin's wriggling had been going on for months, long before the contretemps which was the apparent reason for coming that day. Lying and stealing, like learning difficulties, are ways which children use relatively frequently at Colin's age to signal that they have problems. It was unfortunate perhaps that Mrs Dilley had ignored Colin's lying and stealing. The Dilley household, it transpired, provided the peculiar mixture of a disrupted family structure and over-stimulation due to violence between mother and stepfather which is often found in children with Colin's problems. The doctor discovered later that his previous teacher had many times ignored opportunities to catch Colin out in manifest lies, out of sympathy for Colin's home circumstances. It may not have been a wise decision.

The story of Colin Dilley stops well before the possibility of a solution arises, or even before the nature of the problem is clear.

Quite often a doctor finds himself defining a problem in the only way that suggests a solution—not a strictly logical approach, but at least a practical one. The next issue to consider therefore is the ways in which problems can be solved.

Three ways of solving problems

Dudley (1970) suggests that the answers to three questions indicate the best way of tackling a clinical problems: Can the problem be looked at in such a way that it is not a problem? Can the behaviour which is causing the problem be altered, or its cause eliminated? Or, can the patient's environment be adjusted so that he no longer has the problem?

When dealing with children and their intermediaries, even more than when dealing with other age groups, the general practitioner is rarely fortunate enough to be presented with just one problem, so that solutions from more than one of the three categories must often be considered.

Liquidating a problem

> Mrs Eggleton brought her 3-month-old only child to the well-baby clinic. 'I think Nigel needs circumcising,' she said. She told the doctor that her brother had been circumcised when he was less than a year old and Nigel's foreskin did not seem to retract fully. The doctor explained that the present day view was that there was no need to do anything before the age of 3 to a foreskin which was giving no trouble. He forebore to add that attempts at retraction should be avoided. Mrs Eggleton seemed relieved to hear that her child need not be operated upon and seemed to prepared to consider the problem as liquidated and to pass on to the doctor the responsibility for supervision.

Liquidating a problem does not always mean that a general practitioner is rid of his patient. What happens all too often, to continue the financial metaphor, is that the liquidated problem is taken over by a conglomerate.

> Mrs Finch, an attractive woman who looked four or five years younger than her 26 years, consulted the doctor on the day she registered. She brought with her three children: a 9-year old boy, a 7-year old girl and a robust 2½-year-old little girl. Mrs Finch asked the new doctor a question or two in passing about each of the older children and then took a deep breath. Would the doctor examine the 2½-year-old, Melissa? Melissa, meanwhile, had been systematically destroying the consulting room, around which she charged like a miniature armoured car. Every time Mrs Finch made a half-hearted ineffectual attempt at controlling her, Melissa screamed at her and returned happily to her self-imposed task of mayhem. The doctor could not remember ever seeing a child healthier than Melissa appeared to be. He asked Mrs Finch if the two older children might go into the waiting room. When they did so Melissa immediately stopped her destructive activity and stood literally at her mother's

knee whilst Mrs Finch talked to the doctor. As soon as Mrs Finch paid Melissa the slightest attention, she began her destructive activities again. When Mrs Finch picked her up, Melissa began to scream. The doctor asked what made Mrs Finch feel that Melissa should be examined. 'Because she keeps getting colds.' 'And what about her screaming?' asked the doctor. 'That, too, I suppose,' said Mrs Finch, doubtfully. The doctor said that Melissa appeared to be *too* well and full of energy, but that he would examine her if Mrs Finch wished. Mrs Finch looked at the doctor with a mixture of sadness and despair. An image flashed through the doctor's mind of an object desperately loved but sadly disliked. 'I'm going to ask you what may seem a strange question, Mrs Finch,' he said. 'Was Melissa a planned child?' 'No, she wasn't, but that isn't the trouble. The trouble is that they thought she was an ectopic pregnancy and admitted me to hospital.' Mrs Finch went on to explain how she had been very pleased when the pregnancy proved to be a normal one, but some of the things the doctors had said had led her to believe that her baby would be abnormal, and Melissa did have all these colds, and was very very difficult to handle.

The general practitioner thought that recurrent colds might have been easier to treat!

Changing behaviour or eliminating its cause

The doctor was interrupted during a Friday evening surgery by a telephone request to speak to 32-year-old Ms Green (as she insisted on being called) whose first baby had been delivered fourteen days earlier. The doctor remembered that when she had registered with him she had been six months pregnant and already booked for delivery at a nearby hospital; she had preferred to continue the non-shared care already arranged, and he had seen her only once during the pregnancy about a minor discomfort. She said that she had been home for a few days and was breast-feeding. The baby always had wind after a feed but now it had been screaming for three hours: the doctor could hear it over the telephone.

Within ten minutes the doctor was faced in his surgery by a desperate-looking mother, a lost-looking father and a bright red, yelling baby. The baby, the doctor was told, fed well and opened its bowels regularly but simply did not settle after some of its feeds. It had never screamed for as long as this before. Ms Green undressed the baby completely and the baby continued to scream. The doctor could find nothing wrong, and said so. Ms Green responded by saying that she felt a dreadful failure. The baby had been delivered by forceps under a block. She had held the baby in her arms immediately after delivery: every opportunity for normal bonding had existed. As Ms Green spoke to the doctor the baby quietened. The father then joined in the conversation. Theirs was a regular relationship although they were not married. Could the fact that they were non-Vegan vegetarians cause the breast-fed baby any problems? The doctor felt able to reassure them.

As the conversation proceeded and the baby settled, the doctor became reasonably certain that what lay at the root of the matter was the mother's uncertainty and sense of failure. These problems were exacerbated by what appeared to be a household rule that both parents must look after the baby, not taking it in turns or sharing out their duties but literally passing the he baby back and forth between them as a matter of principle. The doctor talked to the couple about individual babies having individual personalities and about the manner in which the establishment of rituals might be helpful to all three of them. The

interview ended with the baby beginning a different kind of crying (it had not
been fed for more than four hours) and going on to suck hungrily at its mother's
breast.

This anecdote, like most of the others in this chapter, does not
deal with a case completed, but it does illustrate the possibility of
defining a problem in terms of behaviour that can be altered;
organic illness is not excluded and there is no guarantee that it is
not also present. The doctor had only begun to explore the situation: he did not understand yet, for example, the part played by
the parents' deliberate flouting of convention and Ms Green's deep
sense of failure at having a forceps delivery rather than a natural
confinement, or, indeed, her absolute refusal to be addressed as
either 'Mrs' or 'Miss'.

Adjusting the environment
The notion of adjusting the patient's environment so that he no
longer has the problem is particularly attractive in the management
of children because they are presented by intermediaries who may
often seem to the doctor to be producing an environment physically
or emotionally disadvantageous to the child. The technique needs
two cautions: first the intermediary and the doctor must accept that
the child has a problem which is irremediable, at least for the
moment; and secondly, the change of environment may initially
disturb an uneasy equilibrium before things settle down.

> Jimmy Hoadley was 11 years old and an albino. His mother had made
> desperate efforts to provide him with a life as much like that of her other ten
> children as possible. There were, of course, limits to this: it was necessary, for
> instances, for Jimmy to attend a school for the partly-sighted. It was necessary
> also for Jimmy to protect himself against bright sunlight. Despite all her
> efforts Mrs Hoadley found herself shutting off Jimmy from contact with
> children on the newly-built Council housing estate to which the family had
> been moved by sympathetic social workers, because it was nearer to Jimmy's
> school. Mrs Hoadley's new doctor found himself having to provide a great
> deal of support to her so that she allowed Jimmy to play with the children of
> their new neighbourhood. These children, like all children, cruelly highlighted
> Jimmy's physical differences, but as Mrs Hoadley relaxed her protectiveness
> Jimmy became a leader of the other children whilst still taking sensible steps
> to protect himself from strong sunlight.

Collusions of anonymity
Consultations about children are complicated not only by the intermediary, rapid development and bypass mechanisms. They are
affected also by the fear that the very young are more at risk when
physically ill than adolescents or adults are. This fear leads a doctor
to admit a baby to hospital for observation more readily than he

would an adult, and makes him have reservations about relying on a child's verbal story even when this is available. As a consequence, reinforced in particularly by the bypass mechanisms, it is all too easy for a multiplicity of agencies to be involved in attempting to provide care for an individual child and its family. This sharing of responsibility, it has been pointed out by Balint, can lead to 'a collusion of anonymity'. Divided responsibility inevitably, but not always justifiably, reflects a lack of confidence on the part of one or more of those providing the child and family with care. This lack of confidence is not restricted to the care of children, but it does appear in its most flagrant form as a result of the constraints and threats which this task imposes. Balint points out that in a true collusion of anonymity, it seems that no one need feel responsible for what happens as long as 'everybody is trying hard'.

The doctor had had numerous letters from a nearby teaching hospital about them long before he met Miss Isaac and her 18-month-old daughter Linda.
The Isaacs had been told to sign on the doctor's list by the social worker to whom they had been assigned when they moved into the locality. Before giving this instruction, the social worker had telephoned the general practitioner asking permission to do so. When the doctor asked *why* he was being asked the social worker said that Miss Isaac was a manic-depressive and Linda was a very difficult child who was constantly in hospital. The social worker wished Miss Isaac not to have the trauma of being refused admission to a doctor's list because of the predictable difficulties in looking after her.
Hospital letters began to arrive on the general practitioner's desk at a rate of two or three a week. They originated from: gynaecologists, concerning Miss Isaac's irregular periods and intolerance of various versions of the contraceptive pill; the psychiatrist who was monitoring the level of her serum lithium (and presumably her mania); the psychotherapist running the therapy group which Miss Isaac attended—or, more accurately, did not always attend; the paediatrician who was keeping an eye on Linda's development; a variety of paediatric house officers who saw her when she was admitted to hospital; and the dermatologist who was advising on the management of her eczema.
Finally, there were copies of letters from the hospital social worker to the community social worker and from both social workers to a Housing Association, together with the replies.
The doctor was having no trouble acting as the communications centre mentioned earlier in this chapter; his problem was that he never saw Miss Isaac. It seemed to him that the hospital was desperately trying to care for bits of the Isaacs' problems. The gynaecologist seemed frightened that Miss Isaac might fall pregnant again; the community social worker was concerned by Miss Isaac's isolation and lack of friends, especially male friends; the psychiatrist was unhappy that she did not always take her tablets and almost certainly didn't take them at the intervals appropriate for blood-testing; the psychotherapist was moved, at least in part, by the effect on his therapy group of Miss Isaac's irregular attendance; the dermatologist felt that the main problem with Linda's skin was that Miss Isaac didn't obey instructions for its management rigorously or vigorously; the paediatrician, apparently reluctantly, provided Miss Isaac with sedative antihistamines because Linda 'never slept', and Linda appeared to be admitted to the hospital whenever Miss Isaac became concerned about her snuffling, feeding, bowel movements or

sleeplessness. The general practitioner felt that his communication centre was jammed with information and had no trouble thinking in terms of anonymity—he never saw the Isaacs. He wondered, indeed, how they would ever find time to consult him.

Eventually, Miss Isaac did consult him when Linda had a cold. She gave him a picture of her appalling difficulty in making relationships which started at the age of 2 when her mother deserted her. She now had real, and largely insoluble, financial difficulties. Her social difficulties were unlikely to be diminished by the fact that she was a Jewish biochemist, whilst Linda was a curly-topped black delight of a toddler who screamed 'No!' at any approach made by the doctor, but gurgled happily and brought out toys to hand him when he stopped making approaches.

The case of Miss Isaac and Linda has all the characteristics of a 'collusion of anonymity'. Miss Isaac, it proved later, was not the helpless victim of a series of doctors deliberately dodging responsibility; she ran fairly consciously from one doctor to another evoking their sympathy and getting them to relieve her of her responsibilities. It is important for all doctors to realise that a 'collusion of anonymity' is unlikely to be helpful either to the patient or to any of the doctors, and that crises of confidence about the management of families may be properly resolved by the involvement of others only if a clear-cut agreement is established between the patient and all the professionals involved about who is to be primarily responsible.

References

Dudley H A F 1970 The clinical task. Lancer ii: 1352–1354
Balint M 1964 The doctor, his patient and the illness, 2nd edn. Pitman Medical, London pp 69–80

15

The elderly

The elderly now make up about a sixth of the population and see their general practitioners frequently, but their relationships with their doctors may be difficult at first because their experiences have been so different from his. In this chapter we have tried to develop a few generalisations which may be useful to the doctor before he gets to know his elderly patients as individuals.

Parallel services
The range of helpers and services, professional and voluntary, that society now provides for its elderly citizens is enormous. Referring a patient to any of these services needs just as much care and preparation as, for instance, the referral of a young woman for the termination of a pregnancy.

> When the general practitioner broke into Mrs Andrews's local authority flatlet he did so because her equally elderly neighbours had noticed three full bottles of milk outside her door, with no empties. The apartment was icy cold and almost bare, but meticulously tidy. In one corner wrapped up in scanty bedclothes lay the 76-year-old patient. She was too weak to stand, but tried to resist the doctor's effort to unwrap her, crying bitterly when she failed to do so. Though she was lying in a mess of urine and faeces, she seemed alert mentally and not grossly hypothermic; she was clearly deeply ashamed at being found so soiled with excreta. There was no food at all in the flatlet and only a few leaves of tea in the caddy. The milk was outside the door.
> The general practitioner had previously contacted many services for Mrs Andrews, but she had not taken advantage of the many offers that had been made to her; she smiled sweetly, never actually refusing or offending anyone, but never budging either.

The extended family
In most of his contacts with elderly patients, the doctor is looking for medical answers to problems which are demographic and social in origin. A survey of the elderly at home (Hunt 1978) showed that in 1976 0.3% of people in England aged 65 and over were permanently bedfast and that a further 4.2% (more than a quarter of a million people) were permanently confined to their dwellings. In

the six months before the survey, one third of the people questioned had been visited by a doctor, 4.4% by a health visitor, and 7.8% by a district nurse; 9% reported being visited by a doctor as frequently as once a month. These callers not only provide a variety of professional services, they also bring some contact, however brief, with another human being and with events outside the house. For that third of the elderly who live alone this must be particularly important.

Many of the other two-thirds live with close relatives: enjoyed or endured, involved or isolated, in the nearest our society gets to the 'extended family' of other cultures. The following story is a fairly typical one.

> Mrs Barron, aged 83, lived with her youngest daughter Betty, aged 43, and Betty's illegitimate son Bob, aged 22. She had the multiple physical complaints that so often characterise the elderly: the painful and stiff joints of osteo-arthritis; angina which had been relieved by a cardio-selective beta-blocking agent; emphysema and, over the previous ten years, occasional bouts of bronchitis. Mrs Barron used to visit the doctor at intervals, usually with her eldest daughter Barbara, less often with her grandson, Bob, and rarely with Betty.
>
> One day Betty asked the doctor to call on her mother. Mrs Barron, who was in bed, was complaining of aches and pains, a running nose and sore throat. She was afebrile. The doctor decided to prescribe an antibiotic and suggested that it would be better if she were to sit up in a chair during the day. Mrs Barron seemed dismayed and was obviously reluctant to get up—not at all like her usual bustling, active self.
>
> 'What's wrong?' asked the doctor, 'Why do you want to stay in bed?' Mrs Barron avoided the doctor's eye. Betty cut in 'I think she wants me to stay home from work because Barbara has moved away'—a reference to the elder daughter's recent move to a 'better' area a mile and a half away. The doctor thought Betty was quite correct; so obviously, did Mrs Barron, who came as near to blushing as an 83-year-old can. 'Well' said the doctor, 'you can stay at home for the rest of this week, can't you Betty, even if your mother *is* up in a chair?' 'Of course,' replied Betty, and Mrs Barron smiled happily.

Mrs Barron would, the doctor thought, rapidly recover from her 'flu' but a number of questions remained to be answered. How would she cope with the effects of Barbara's move? How would she manage the shopping now she couldn't stop at Barbara's for a rest on the way? How would she be able to ask for help in the house from Betty when *she* had always given Betty help, and when Betty was the breadwinner? To add a new piece of information, what did Mrs Barron make of the fact that her grandson had recently been bound over for exposing himself indecently to the very next-door neighbour who might otherwise have provided a little help with the shopping?

A memory bank
It is probable that Mrs Barron found today's attitudes to her grandson's behaviour as incomprehensible as the behaviour itself. Despite her old-fashioned mores, Mrs Barron had been able, even after her husband's death 15 years earlier, to exercise the function of 'village elder', and to be of value as a living memory bank for her descendants. This role has been taken away from most elderly people by the rapid changes in our society and its technology; they have been robbed of a prime function and given little or nothing in its place, turning them into useless appendages to their community.

In Mrs Barron's case society may have been wise to forgo her particular family skills. She had another daughter, who suffered from epilepsy and episodes of paranoia and had been deserted by her husband. There was a son of 15 who was truanting persistently from school and who had appeared in court several times for 'taking and driving away' motor cars. Nevertheless, it was probably the continued use of her acquired skills and knowledge that had kept Mrs Barron so active and young-looking despite her multiple physical disabilities.

Social disengagement
Physical deterioration eventually prevents people from making the simple minor adjustments by means of which they remain in reasonably stable emotional equilibrium, and it sets in well before senescence or even retirement. Older workers tend to use and be used to older machines and older methods, so that the introduction of new machines and new methods usually means that younger workers have to be recruited. When the older techniques are abandoned there may be no occupational role for older workers at all, because re-training them is uneconomical and difficult. They are as competent as younger ones in jobs which require simple repetitive movements or paced and discontinuous muscular activity, but it is often socially unacceptable to have them doing the 'heavy' work while younger employees carry out the 'lighter', power-assisted activities.

A similar consideration affects clerical jobs. Older people seem more likely to abandon problems with which they are not familiar and cannot deal by pattern recognition; they tend to settle for approximate rather than precise solutions. Unfortunately, it is in positions of management acquired by experience rather than by diplomas that accuracy is more important than approximation when decisions have to be made. A parallel in everyday life is familiar:

the elderly person who walks briskly to the kerb of a pedestrian crossing, dithers a moment, then dashes into the path of oncoming traffic.

Strategies for adjustment

In the face of functional impairment and social pressures, the ageing individual has to find a way of adapting and coping.

People come to terms with life in a variety of ways, but preferably in ways which evolve from their earlier patterns of behaviour—tactics for survival that have been proven during their earlier life. Elderly people usually become more fixed in their attitudes and their personality traits become more obvious; perhaps they see less need to camouflage them. Eccentricity can be endearing but bizarre behaviour disturbs other people. D. B. Bromley (1966), in a Pelican Original entitled *The Psychology of Human Ageing*, offers descriptions of five strategies for adjustment which may be adopted in old age; they are based on an American study by Suzanne Reichard and her colleagues Florine Livson and P. G. Petersen. The five strategies are: 'Constructiveness'; 'Dependency'; 'Defensiveness'; 'Hostility'; and 'Self-hate'.

Socially acceptable strategies

Constructiveness and dependency

> Mr Collins was aged 75 and his wife was 72; the doctor had looked after them for more than ten years. Mrs Collins had always been a tense anxious woman whose 'palpitations' were eventually replaced by a moderate angina and mild high-output failure. During his wife's gradual deterioration in health Mr Collins preserved himself well and kept his part-time job at the heavy vehicles factory where he had worked all his life. He could be relied upon to make a common-sense but concerned and perceptive response to his wife's anxious comments. He joked occasionally about the failure of the computer to replace him completely as a store-manager, and how the firm still needed him part-time to get the job done properly.
>
> One evening the doctor received an agonised call from Mrs Collins to the effect that her husband was dying. The doctor found him with both lungs full of fluid, a high fever, and just enough breath to murmur through his blue lips that he was 'sorry to be a nuisance'. Mr Collins was admitted to hospital and Mrs Collins went to stay with her son (a head master) and daughter-in-law some miles away in a new and expensive extra-urban housing development. When Mr Collins was discharged from the District General Hospital he manifested the multiple pathology of old age. His cardiac failure was well compensated, but the diuretics had revealed difficulty in micturition which had in turn led to a diagnosis of early malignant change in his prostate—effectively but embarassingly controlled by oestrogens.
>
> Mr Collins and his wife took up their lives again and used to visit the general practitioner monthly for prescriptions which Mr Collins would dictate in detail. At one such consultation, six months after Mr Collins's discharge,

the doctor thought that Mr and Mrs Collins both seemed rather depressed, and said so to them. Mr Collins took a deep breath, 'Well, you see, doctor, my son wants us to move nearer him.' The doctor made no comment. It seemed an obvious and sensible suggestion and Mr Collins was obviously a sensible man. Mr Collins went on to explain that the sale of his pleasant house and garden would not bring in enough money to buy them similar accommodation in the area in which his son now lived. He and his wife still led a fairly active social life; they felt they had made all the adjustments that they wanted to make, and didn't want to make any more. 'Yes,' chimed in Mrs Collins, 'we've cut down our activities to those we can cope with. We couldn't do with making new friends as well.'

Mr Collins seems to exemplify the strategy Reichard terms *constructiveness*. He had accepted the facts of old age, and was self-sufficient within the limits of his health and circumstances. His interests were well-developed and showed continuity with his earlier life. Mrs Collins on the other hand seems to exemplify *dependency*. Acceptable socially, it is found in fairly well integrated individuals who are prepared to rely upon others. The two strategies complement each other and were well suited to the Collinses. Certainly the couple seemed to have followed together a sensible process of social disengagement. Their son may have seen the move as a way of making more help available to them; they saw it as likely to precipitate their helplessness.

The doctor discussed things with the Collinses a little longer and terminated the consultation with an agreement that they would not move until all three of them, together, had agreed it was necessary. Further, the couple could use the doctor's authority in argument against the suggestion of their well-intentioned son.

Socially unacceptable strategies

Disengaging is essential as people get older, but it should not go so far as to exclude activities that provide human contact and human interest. In trying to help patients to achieve a sensible compromise between disengagement and activity doctors undertake a most important task. All too often disengagement is allowed to becomes a negative process which increasingly isolates an elderly person from the company which stimulates him, and offers him no alternative but to engage in pastimes which hold no attraction for him. Finding the right balance is one of the commonest problems facing doctors who practise in 'retirement' towns: so many of their patients are those ageing migrants who are the refugees and displaced people of our society. One use of the relationship between doctor and patient is in helping avoid unwise decisions of the sort that were nearly forced upon the Collinses. Not all patients, however, have personalities as attractive and co-operative as the Collinses, nor are they as able to develop strategies of disengagement as successful and acceptable as theirs.

Defensiveness

Mrs Andrews, whom the doctor found hypothermic and malnourished in her old-person's flatlet, illustrates the strategy of *defensiveness*. People like her seem to be frightened of the dependency and relative inactivity of old age, and have a pessimistic outlook. Conscious of a deterioration that they are at pains to deny, they refuse the help of younger people. The strategy becomes socially unacceptable when it causes the kind of horrific consequences that Mrs Andrews suffered.

Hostility

For some people, resentment at getting old becomes almost malignant, and they are often terrified of dying. They do not become depressed, but move instead towards paranoia, and are jealous of younger people.

Self-hate

Reichard and her colleagues describe a category of elderly people who accept that they are ageing, but regard their progressive disability as some kind of punishment which they deserve. They are depressed in that they are gloomy and flat in mood, but they do not appear to worry about death nor to fear it: indeed they seem to welcome the prospect, though they do not usually consider killing themselves.

It may be that this group of self-hating patients accounts for the relatively high rate of prescribing of anti-depressant drugs to the elderly as a whole. Reluctance on the part of the doctor to enter into a psychotherapeutic relationship with elderly patients probably plays a part too.

Intellectual impairment

Severe intellectual impairment of the elderly, or dementia, is a relatively infrequent occurrence in general practice, but patients who use a hostile strategy for social disengagement may be judged by others to exhibit some of the characteristics of dementia.

Mrs Davis was 77 when her husband first called the doctor. She had a roaring pneumonia, but her one concern was that she should not be sent to hospital where she was sure she would die or be killed. She said that she was 69 but that her husband believed her to be 61; he certainly seemed unintelligent enough to make the success of her deception credible. Mrs Davis recovered from her pneumonia at home.

Fifteen months later Mrs Davis's downstairs neighbour asked the doctor to visit because Mrs Davis had become very forgetful, and was defaecating in places other than the shared lavatory on the mezzanine floor; she was falling about and spending a lot of her time in bed. When the doctor arrived, Mrs Davis seemed very much her usual self. She denied all the accusations and became very angry when the neighbour, who was much younger, repeated them. The neighbour left in a huff. Mrs Davis then told the doctor that she hadn't always been as well as she was today. She said that her neighbour wanted her rooms and was poisoning her; the doctor had been called so that she would be sent into hospital and killed. The doctor felt very puzzled. He tried assessing Mrs Davis's orientation in time and space with the usual questions, and her intellectual ability by asking her to do simple sums based on her shopping. She had no difficulties with either sort of assessment.

The doctor called in the neighbour again and asked if she could date Mrs Davis's deterioration from any particular event. 'Yes', she said, 'from when your locum called when Mrs Davis had pneumonia again.' The doctor looked back at Mrs Davis's records. She had been visited during the doctor's holiday and given a tetracycline, a cough linctus and some syrup of choral. When the doctor asked Mrs Davis if she still had any of the cough medicine the locum had prescribed, he was presented with a clear syrup with a bitter taste which, she said, was wonderful in stopping her cough from keeping her awake. It was so good that she used it during the day too. The doctor replaced it with simple linctus and there was no more problem about her behaviour. She had confused the linctus with the sedative, not because of a fault on the doctor's part, but because she had complained of coughing at night and had naturally assumed that the medicine to be taken at night was for her cough.

The effects of ageing are greater upon short-term recall than they are on long-term recall. They make new ideas difficult to grasp but leave unaffected the ability to apply old concepts to new facts. Mrs Davis's reasoning was logically impeccable, if only she hadn't forgotten what she had been told.

Prevention

Many doctors seem unable, if not unwilling, to talk to elderly people in the way they do to people nearer their own age. This social difficulty is compounded by beliefs stemming from psychoanalysis about older people's inability to change—and particularly unfortunate when the patient's problems stem from a 'self-hating' strategy that could have been converted to something more constructive and socially acceptable.

Mrs Edge was 71 when her own general practitioner retired and she was issued with a 'new' one. When she met him she was therefore not suffering from the effects of having moved house or of having had a difference with her old doctor in the way most new patients are.

She had a mouse-like appearance and her mood was flat, but she was in good health. She consulted her new doctor a week after her transfer to ask for more of her blood-pressure tablets. The doctor found her blood pressure to be 210/115, and thought that the reserpine she had been taking for 18 years was probably unnecessary. He weaned her off the drug over ten weeks, by which time her blood pressure was 200/100 and she said that she felt much better in herself. She agreed to come back for a further check a few weeks later. In the interval the doctor reviewed Mrs Edge's records back to 1937, in which year she had consulted five times; she had consulted five times in 1938, six in 1939, 26 in 1940, five in 1941, nine in 1942, and so on throughout the years, averaging 15 consultations a year since 1951. The general practitioner wondered if he had been wise to interfere with what has been called 'a peaceful repeat prescription' (Balint et al 1970).

Mrs Edge kept her review appointment and said she was very well; she felt a bit of a fraud, and didn't like bothering the doctor. The doctor remained silent. He had all these ill people to see, didn't he, continued Mrs Edge, and here she was so well. He had been very kind but she didn't like bothering him.

The doctor took a calculated risk.

'Mrs Edge,' he said, 'whenever someone says that they don't like bothering me I wonder if they are really saying that they feel they're not worth bothering about.'

'How right you are, doctor.' replied Mrs Edge. 'I've never felt anything but worthless. I always think I'm tackling things the wrong way, although usually I'm not. I haven't any children because I didn't marry until I was nearly forty—I could never believe that anyone would really want me.'

Mrs Edge went on to describe how this feeling of worthlessness had developed from her childhood experiences and had been reinforced by events during her teens and young adulthood.

'You won't believe this doctor, but I sit in my armchair, sometimes, and cry because I feel so worthless. My husband is very good about it and cuddles me and tells me of course I'm worthwhile, but it doesn't help for long.'

Mrs Edge stopped and looked up timidly at the doctor who asked after a lengthy pause. 'What do you want me to say, Mrs Edge?' Mrs Edge hung her head. After another pause the general practitioner said 'I think that you should come to see me again in two weeks.'

Mrs Edge described a lifetime of low self-esteem, if not quite self-hate. Whether or not it might be possible to modify her way of coping with life is arguable, but it seems unarguable that an attempt many years earlier to recognise it as the reason for her frequent surgery attendances might have led her to a more contented old age.

Trying to identify coping behaviours, and making predictions about the strategies of adaptation to which they will lead, places yet another responsibility upon the doctor, but the story of Mrs Edge suggests that it may be worthwhile. Enough drugs are necessary for treating the diseases of old age without using them to treat the elderly patient's lifestyle too.

References

Hunt A 1978 The elderly at home. Office of Population Censuses and Surveys, HMSO, London

Balint M, Hunt J, Joyce R, Marinker M L, Woodcock J 1970 Treatment or diagnosis—a study of repeat prescriptions in general practice. Tavistock Publications, London

16

A matter of confidence

The point has been made that if direct questions are asked by the doctor the information obtained will be limited to answers to those questions; with an open-ended approach the patient is more likely to talk about the difficulties which really brought him to the consultation.

Throughout this book it has been assumed that the patient will confide in the doctor if the doctor shows sufficient interest. This assumption depends upon another assumption by the patient: that what is said to the doctor will be treated as a professional confidence and will go no further without the patient's permission. There has been increasing publicity about breaches in the assumed confidentiality of information given to doctors. If the patient cannot rely upon his confidences being confidential he will not have the confidence to confide; but if the doctor does as we have suggested, and encourages patients to give him information about matters which are not strictly medical, he must increase his own difficulties in keeping it confidential.

A legal obligation

Mrs Argyle, a 42-year-old patient whom the doctor had often treated for emotional problems, came complaining of anxiety, and immediately launched into the reason for her visit. Her son, aged 17, had been accused of breaking and entering an empty house and with some companions performing acts of vandalism.

'We have given the police a statement which gives the boy an alibi, but we were telling lies and I know he really did it. I don't understand why he did. Would you see him and speak to him?'

Mrs Argyle had told the doctor directly that she had made a false statement to the police intending to pervert the course of justice. Some lawyers would hold that such direct evidence should be passed on to the police even though the mother self-evidently expected the doctor to treat what she had said as 'in confidence'. What Mrs Argyle had said was the real truth about her son's behaviour was only at second-hand, that is, 'hearsay' evidence, and placed no legal obligations upon the doctor. When, later, the 17-year-old himself consulted the doctor and volunteered that he was in fact guilty as accused the doctor's difficulties would be seen by some lawyers to have been compounded: especially since in their role as expert witnesses doctors are given greater leeway by the Court in reporting as evidence what patients have said to them during consultations. One argument a doctor could use is that in the case of Mrs Argyle he was not an expert witness, but many doctors feel entitled to use as a criterion the gravity of the offence admitted, striking a balance between responsibility as a doctor and responsibility as a citizen when deciding whether or not to maintain a patient's confidence. But what if the offence for which an alibi was being given had been murder? It is not sufficient to say: 'I will ignore my legal obligations here, but if the matter were more serious then I would feel obliged to break confidentiality.'

Moral judgements and the public weal
There is an important, even if not sharply definable, distinction to be made between moral judgements, whether within or without the law, and judgements about predictable material risk to the community. If a patient admits to an illegal action the doctor cannot decide where his duty lies by reference to his own personal standards of behaviour or severity. He is not a judge. He is, however, in a position to have the patient consider, within the context of the doctor-patient relationship, what action the latter will take. If the patient is unable, or refuses, to move towards a legally acceptable decision, the doctor is faced, inexorably, with a duty to society at large that takes precedence over his professional ethic. At the same time, if there are frequent breaches of confidence, confidences will cease to be made; the law will be no better defended and society will be much the poorer in the quality of its medical care.

When on the other hand, a predictable material risk to the community presents itself, as in the familiar cases of the typhoid carrier or the epileptic train driver, the doctor can adjudicate between the requirements of the doctor-patient relationship and those of the community, which in such circumstances he can see as a congregation of patients. Fortunately such situations are too rare to create a major difficulty. Any extension of the laws requiring doctors to notify certain diseases to the authorities might enlarge this difficulty, but then at least the obligation would be public (and, in a democracy, the people's will) and implicit in the contract offered by the doctor before the consultation.

Another way in which a doctor, especially in general practice, may find himself in difficulties over confidentiality and crime is to accept unquestioningly that criminal behaviour is illness simply because it is deviant. A sharp distinction must be drawn between a criminal action and the distress it causes to the apprehended culprit.

Mr Billings, aged 22, slumped in his chair and looked at the ground. 'I'm terribly depressed, doctor.' When encouraged to go further he explained that he had broken into an off-licence two nights before and had been caught by the police. After being charged, he had appeared at the Magistrate's Court next morning when the case had been adjourned. 'You're not depressed,' said the doctor, 'You're miserable, and you're a thief.'

This unorthodox approach made a sharp distinction between the crime and the patient's mood; it was one which the patient seemed able to appreciate, because he was immediately happy to discuss his motives for the theft with the doctor.

Three temptations
Problems about confidentiality are not confined to legal issues.

The doctor who encourages his patients to talk freely about non-medical matters meets three further dilemmas. First, he may feel that a particular person is the source of the patient's difficulties and he may wish to speak to that person utilising information obtained from his interview with the patient. Secondly, he may feel he would like to alter other people's behaviour towards his patient, not because they themselves are unreasonable but because the patient's condition would be improved by an alteration. Thirdly, the patient's story may sound so bizarre that he needs to test it against reality by discussion with the other people involved.

In any of these three situations the doctor may be able to avoid breaking confidence by obtaining the patient's permission to speak; but it will be clear to practising doctors that to seek such permission is often an ultimatum which says: 'If you won't give me permission I will not be able to continue treating you.' Nothing could be more destructive to a co-operative relationship.

Of the three situations described above, the first was touched on in the chapter dealing with the Family, where it was observed that the temptation to agree with the present patient to treat an absent one should usually be avoided, since it is almost always a strategy to enable both doctor and patient to avoid facing certain painful aspects of reality.

The second situation is one which does not often cause any real difficulty because it is usually the patient who requests the action. The doctor's main concern may be to satisfy himself that he is not just being manipulated.

The third situation, where the objective truth of the patient's statement is doubted, can be a real snare for the unwary doctor. Whereas in the first situation he was tempted to avoid treating the patient as ill by defining someone else's behaviour as the cause of a normal reaction, here he is tempted to define the patient as ill because he doubts the truth of the patient's beliefs. If the doctor hopes to use his relationship with the patient therapeutically, he has to accept that he must work with whatever the patient believes to be true, and the only checks he can apply are those that arise from inconsistencies within the patient's story.

Internal and external reality
The issue of internal and external reality is of the utmost importance in considering whether or not the doctor should be compelled by law to reveal a patient's confidences. It is not the doctor's task to seek external reality, and the emotions released in a consultation may so colour the patient's version of an incident as to make it inconsistent even with his own previous account of the same happening. To report any one version out of context in a Court may be more dangerously misleading than to remain silent. In the United States there is more legal protection for both patient and doctor than there is in this country, some two thirds of States having some statutory provision for 'testimonial privilege'. In both countries, and throughout the Commonwealth, the trend is towards greater legal recognition of the rights of privacy.

Twin errors
Difficulties over confidences most often arise from the temptation to use information given by one member of a family when dealing with another member.

Mrs Campbell, aged 45, had multiple physical illnesses but usually consulted her doctor to complain about her husband. She would say that he showed her no sympathy when she was ill, insisted upon her doing things like decorating the house though she was physically unable to, rarely spoke to her except to give an order, and continued even through her ill health to insist upon his sexual rights.

Their son, aged 23, developed a duodenal ulcer, and told the doctor how he felt a need to protect his mother from his father. He had fallen in love and wanted to get married, but then he would have to leave mother alone with father 'And you know how he treats her, doctor!' The doctor agreed, 'Yes, I do.' Only later did the doctor discover that the father was far from being the unfeeling brute his wife held him to be; she was manipulating her son heavily to try to stop him from leaving home.

The doctor had committed the twin errors of accepting the patient's statements as external reality without further checks, and of revealing his knowledge of the mother's confidences to the son. (Whether or not the mother would have approved of this breach of confidence is irrelevant.) Both errors, and much subsequent ill health and unhappiness for the family, would have been avoided if the doctor had abided by the rules of confidentiality and answered the son instead: 'Why don't you tell me about it?'

Informed consent

The idea that the doctor's seeking permission from a patient to break a confidence may be taken by the patient as an ultimatum can be extended to the matter of consent by patients in general practice to being included in research projects. The subject is difficult, but just as fostering a good relationship depends upon encouraging the patient to talk about anything he thinks is relevant, so the existence of such a relationship demands that the doctor should state explicitly that refusal to take part in research in no way threatens it. The best way of making this clear may be for consent to be sought by a third person, with the guarantee that the doctor will know neither who has been approached nor who has refused. This step can usually be built without difficulty into a double-blind trial. When it comes to agreeing to video or audio recordings the problems of informed consent is of a different order. The patient is in the position of the little girl whose mother asks her 'Why don't you think before you speak?' only to receive the reply 'How can I know what I'm going to say till I say it!' Permission to record must be sought before a recording is made and the guarantee given that if permission *is* given, further permission will be sought to retain the recording after the consultation is over. Again a third person—perhaps a receptionist—should do the asking on both occasions.

A personal practical code

The consulting-room is as confidential as the confessional, but for the doctor there are no rigid religious dicta to turn to, or to beset him. To use his relationships with his patients in diagnosis, therapy and prevention, the general practitioner must develop his own practical code for the preservation of confidences; he will need it in almost all his consultations.

17

Treating the cause

The idea that a doctor's first task is to 'find the cause' was instilled into us as medical students. Sets of symptoms were supposed to make us think about which disease was causing them and then about what was causing the disease.

The value of a causal approach is obvious when removing the cause removes the effects, or when it can be used prospectively to define criteria for successful treatment, but a retrospective search for 'the cause' in general practice can be curiously irrelevant. It is usually too elusive to pin down or too difficult to remove, and removing it does not guarantee that the effects will disappear. In any case, the general practitioner's first task is to understand what his patient's behaviour means, and before he can be sure that he does he may have to test a great many assumptions.

Searching for 'the cause' leads inevitably to the labelling of symptoms as either organic or psychogenic, and indirectly to the recurrent controversy about whether the general practitioner's role should be scientific or pastoral. This misses the point entirely—he is part of the patient's environment, affecting the patient both directly and indirectly, and his actions weave themselves into the fabric of the patient's life.

This is not to say that what he does is unimportant—he can do a great deal of good and a great deal of harm, as the concepts of 'observer interference' and 'optimum intervention' emphasise.

Observer interference

It is recognised in the basic sciences that observing a phenomenon of itself alters the phenomenon, and in medicine no consultation with a conscious patient can ever be merely diagnostic: it always has some effects on the patient's subsequent feelings and behaviour. Since the doctor can rarely limit his actions to those whose effects he can predict, he needs some idea of how the patient sees his actions.

Mrs Ashworth, a 40-year-old woman fairly well-known to the doctor, complained of tiredness, waking up early and other symptoms which seemed to justify a diagnosis of mild depression. He was very rushed that evening, and prescribed an anti-depressant without more ado. He briefly mentioned the side-effects of the drug and also the time-lag before it could be expected to work, and arranged to see her two weeks later.

When she came back she was as depressed as before. She said that she had not taken the tablets properly because they made her feel so peculiar. The doctor thought that his hurry in the first consultation might have played a part in this and made it obvious that she now had his whole attention.

He learned that she remembered her mother as a terrible nagger and her father as a man who never had time for anyone except himself. There was no love in the house, either between her parents or between them and any of the children. She had been determined that her own children would have a happier home. The doctor recalled that she had had to take her son to the Child Guidance Clinic recently for some minor delinquency and commented that perhaps that was why this episode had been so hard on her. Mrs Ashworth burst into tears and said she felt such a failure. After all her ideas about creating a loving family she was being hateful to everyone and her son was having to see a psychiatrist.

It seemed as though Mrs Ashworth had seen the hurried prescription in terms of her relationship with her parents—a present to get rid of her rather than to show love. Perhaps she had heard the instruction to come back in two weeks as meaning 'stay away for a fortnight', and the nature of the prescription itself as a further confirmation of her failure.

The placebo effect is a well-documented phenomenon and is a clear demonstration of observer interference, since the essential ingredient seems to be the belief which the patient carries away with him about the preparation. There may well be a 'negative placebo' effect too, and Mrs Ashworth may have been suffering from it. Perhaps the high failure rate of psychotropic drugs in general is due to the way in which they are presented.

If the doctor does not know how the patient views the medication given him, he cannot know what effect it will have.

Optimum intervention

When the doctor understands why a patient has consulted him he may find that more than one course of action is open to him, and this is especially true when the patient has been given a chance to enlarge on the presenting complaint. An optimum intervention is one in which the doctor strikes the best balance he can between short-term and long-term considerations. Short-term considerations are about immediate relief, long-term considerations are about the ways in which his actions may affect the patient's future life, often in areas that are nothing to do with medicine.

Mrs Berwick, a new patient aged 50, was complaining of abdominal pain. After being a widow for ten years she had married again just three months earlier. Six months before that, with no thought of re-marriage in her mind, she had booked herself the 'holiday of a lifetime' for which she had been saving up over many years. The holiday was due to begin in two weeks' time, but for good business reasons her new husband could not go with her. At first he had said that of course she must go, but now he seemed resentful and was behaving childishly. What could she do about the terrible pains she was getting?

What was the cause of the pain? Was it because she could not make up her mind? Why was her husband so unreasonable? Did he not trust her? She had offered to do whatever he wanted, but he had said that she must decide for herself. They were both very worried about her pains.

The doctor found no physical abnormality other than increased bowel sounds. He decided to prescribe an antispasmodic in the hope that this would reduce her physical discomfort, and made no special comment as he handed her the prescription.

Mrs Berwick's pain had offered the possibility of cancelling the holiday without losing either face or money; it had also aroused some concern in her husband. The doctor had no idea what the effect on her marriage might be if he diagnosed her mental conflict as the cause of the pain. He could see that the holiday and the pain were both forcing her to examine her relationship with her husband; relieving the pain would probably not stop this process, but most of the other actions he could think of probably would. On balance, he thought he had made the optimum intervention for the moment.

Conclusion
These are cautionary tales, reminding us that the doctor himself is still probably the most important part of the treatment, as Balint emphasised so many years ago. He administers himself through his relationship with his patients, and the effects may have a very long half-life indeed.

Summaries of the case-histories

CHAPTER 1—AN INTRODUCTION

Mrs Avis p. 1

A girl with severe facial scarring and serious personal problems who was referred to a dermatologist for possible planing of the skin, while the general practitioner continued to deal with her emotional difficulties. Out-patient treatment proving ineffective, the registrar wanted to admit her so that a social worker could talk to her—his concept of 'whole-person care'.

Mrs Bellamy p. 2

A woman who, after a period of infertility, had an abnormal baby and became depressed. Many kinds of outside agency might have been helpful to her, but the general practitioner decided not to call them in until he understood her better.

Mr Cramble p. 4

An elderly patient who was clearly ill but who gave a very vague history. He refused to go to hospital, but when seen at home the next day by a surgeon gave him a classical history of gall-stone colic.

CHAPTER 2—THE RELATIONSHIP

Mr Abel p. 6

An American who did not understand the British medical system and was upset when the consultation did not go as he was expecting it to.

Mrs Bates p. 6

A woman whose previous experience with general practitioners led her into mistaken beliefs about her new doctor that puzzled him.

Miss Cable p. 7

A woman who had poor expectations of general practitioners as a result of past experiences. When the new doctor behaved differently there was a good outcome.

Mrs Dale p. 7

A woman whose behaviour did not conform to the doctor's expectations, leaving him annoyed and inhibited.

Mrs Eames p. 8
A woman who was going bald and was not consoled by being told that tests showed nothing abnormal.

Mr & Mrs Fair p. 8
A couple who could not understand the failure of medical science to deal with the simple problem of their infertility.

Mr Greaves p. 9
A man whose clear but mistaken beliefs about the way the body works created some confusion.

Mrs Halliwell p. 10
A woman who was frightened that she had a cerebral tumour. She interpreted the symptoms of her anxiety as signs of the tumour.

Mr Imber p. 10
A man with both physical and emotional problems. The doctor chose to deal with the former first and controlled the consultation accordingly.

Mr Jarrett p. 11
An angry man who misunderstood the doctor's refusal to give him the analgesics he wanted, seeing it as arbitrarily authoritarian. He was satisfied when given a rational explanation.

CHAPTER 3—ASSUMPTIONS

Wendy Acheson p. 18
A girl whose assumptions about men and marriage led her to accept repeated venereal infection from her husband in a way that amazed her doctor.

Michael Burford p. 19
A young man whose assumptions about how to behave when angry were so different from those of his employer that he thought he was ill and left his job.

Mrs Charnley p. 19
A woman whose assumptions about when babies should be clean were at odds with those of her doctor. He mishandled the situation and lost a patient.

Mr Duleep p. 19
A Sikh who assumed that his nocturnal emissions were a sign of illness. His doctor recognised the cultural difficulty and was able to reassure him tactfully.

Mrs Easton p. 20
A woman who took the diagnosis of nits in her son's hair as an accusation of neglect. The doctor dispelled her anger by telling her that his own child had suffered from the same condition.

Mrs French p. 21
A woman who believed that her symptoms were organic while her doctor thought them emotional in origin. They failed to negotiate any common ground.

Jenny Garner p. 21
A woman who wanted to carry on taking a high dose of hypnotics. The doctor believed he could wean her off them given time and negotiated a compromise with her.

Mrs Hillman p. 22
An old lady who was glad to talk about her loneliness but not to acknowledge it as the real reason for her consultation. The doctor helped her to save face by treating the cold with which she presented.

Mrs Illingworth p. 22
A woman who presented with nocturnal cramps and made no mention of her suicidal intentions. The doctor discovered her depression fortuitously and she decided not to kill herself, though she said nothing of this either.

Mr Jamieson p. 23
A man who was disturbed by evidence of his body failing him and unable to accept a diagnosis of depression because he interpreted it as meaning that his mind was also failing.

Mrs King p. 24
A woman who was seriously frightened of hereditary psychiatric illness. The problem came to light because the doctor responded to her gynaecological presenting symptoms in an open-ended way.

Mr Logan p. 25
A man who assumed that treatment for his backache would be lengthy and mean time off work. He was baffled when given immediate relief by manipulation.

Mrs Martin p. 25
A woman who assumed that the doctor would give her advice about her marital problems and was frustrated by his counselling approach.

Mr Nugent p. 25
A man who believed he needed a tonic and could not accept the doctor's refusal to give him one.

Cheryl Ogden p. 26
A male trainee, unable to make a diagnosis for this attractive girl, assumed that he had failed medically because he had done no more than talk to her in a way they both enjoyed.

Mrs Phillips p. 27
A woman who asked her doctor to visit though she knew her child had chicken pox and what to do about it. Whatever her assumptions about the need for a call, they were apparently shared by the doctor.

CHAPTER 4—UNDERSTANDING AND INSIGHT

Mrs Arden p. 28
The doctor's surprise at this woman's behaviour implied beliefs about normal sexual activity which prevented her from talking about her unhappy marriage.

Mrs Blaise p. 29
A woman who suppressed clinically important information because she wanted to fulfill a social obligation. The doctor reached the right diagnosis as a result of observing her appearance.

Mrs Corless p. 29
A woman who suppressed information because of her fear of cancer. The doctor discovered it after observing her reluctance to leave when her presenting symptoms had been dealt with.

Mrs Daiches p. 30
An incidental moral judgement by the doctor led this midwife to conceal her true parity and resulted in an unsuitable home confinement being arranged. Her anger, concealed for a long time, was eventually taken out on a different doctor.

Mary Ellard p. 31
A child who was anxious about her mother and refused to go to school. She got her mother to sanction this by having symptoms that made her mother anxious.

Mr Followes p. 31
A man who did not see a connection between his eczema flaring up and his unwillingness to face problems at work. The doctor witheld any easy interpretation because he felt he did not know the patient well enough.

Mrs Griggs p. 32
The doctor suspected that this woman was witholding information when she tried to influence him by behaviour that was first promotive and then evocative.

Mrs Hazel p. 33
A woman who was willing to talk about her problems only when the doctor said that he knew there must be something wrong but that he would not try to push her to discuss them.

Miss Ibbotson p. 34
A girl whose consultations with the doctor had always been bilaterally flirtatious. When she needed help seriously it was difficult for them to break the tradition.

Mrs Jackson p. 35
A woman who was trying to hide her marital problems but offered a clue by making a slip of the tongue.

Mrs Knowles p. 35
A woman who indicated how irrelevant her presenting problem had been by forgetting to pick up the prescription after her real problems had been discussed.

Miss Long p. 35
A patient who offered many vague symptoms and denied that there were any stresses in her life. The impasse was broken only when the doctor confessed himself confused.

Peter Mason p. 35
A boy with recurrent abdominal pain. A clue to its cause was seen by the doctor in part of the history which he interpreted symbolically.

Mrs Nettle p. 36
A woman who had a lengthy consultation about her children and, as she was leaving, came to the real point with a 'By the way, doctor. . . .'

Mrs Oakes p. 36
A woman who attended the surgery frequently but without satisfaction to herself or the doctor. Eventually she was allowed to talk freely; no diagnosis emerged but it improved the relationship in a way that made the future seem brighter.

CHAPTER 5—THE DOCTOR'S FEELINGS—A SIXTH SENSE

James Arthur p. 39
A boy with acne whose mother's behaviour made the doctor angry because he had not got over feelings about his own mother's behaviour when he had acne himself.

Miss Buxton p. 41
A woman who found help in bearing her misfortunes from the doctor's encouraging manner. When he became visibly depressed by his inability to do anything more for her she found the strength to comfort him.

Mrs Cummings p. 41
A patient who persistently irritated her doctor. He resented her continual implications that he was to blame for not being able to cure her; when he explained how he felt the effect was surprisingly constructive.

Mr Dodgson p. 42
A man for whose symptoms the doctor could never find an explanation. He was able to understand how the doctor's behaviour came to be conditioned by expectations of disappointment because of his own experiences, and their relationship improved.

Mrs Entwistle p. 43
A woman whose aura of misery made the doctor so uncomfortable that he always tried to end her consultations about her children and persistently failed to notice that she was in pain.

Mrs Farmer p. 43
A man whose complaints made the doctor feel depressed. This was the only overt diagnostic pointer to the patient's depression.

Amanda Garson p. 44
A girl whose attractiveness was difficult for the doctor to cope with. This proved to be a clue to understanding her problems.

Mrs Hill p. 44

A woman who, when anxious about her child, would skilfully arouse her doctors' professional anxieties in unjustifiable ways. This invariably made them angry, and it was only when one was able to see her behaviour as a symptom to be explored that things improved.

CHAPTER 6—EMPATHY AND SYMPATHY

Mr Abernethy p. 48

Suddenly recognising the despair in this man's voice when he made one of his regular visits for his wife's prescription gave the doctor an unexpected insight, which was followed up in more conventional ways to good effect.

Robert Black p. 49

The doctor found this boy sullen and unco-operative until he suddenly realised that he was being seen as no more than an extension of parental authority. He was able to use this insight constructively.

Mr Coghill p. 49

A man who found the doctor's genuine sympathy for his impossibly difficult situation a help in carrying on.

Mrs Drabble p. 50

A woman who enlisted the doctor's sympathy in her marital problems; it was only when a different doctor challenged her to look at her own part in the problems that any progress was possible.

Mrs Edwards p. 50

A doctor who sympathised too quickly about events in this woman's life prevented her from telling him what she really felt about them. This made it impossible for him to help her with her subsequent symptoms.

Mrs Franks p. 51

A difficult patient who was one day given a chance to talk fully. The doctor did nothing other than listen carefully, but this improved subsequent consultations. He displayed not sympathy, but what is often called a 'sympathetic approach'.

CHAPTER 7—FOSTERING A RELATIONSHIP

Mrs Childs p. 53

This patient's story unfolds over a period of two years. For most of this time the doctor was not allowed to be directly helpful; instead he acted on his belief that she needed to experience the particular kind of relationship which he tried to provide. The approach showed some promise in that she became less defensive.

CHAPTER 8—DISHONEST RELATIONSHIPS

Mr Anthony p. 63
A man who was overweight and short of breath on exertion but took no notice of his general practitioner's advice, denigrated the opinion of the cardiologist to whom he insisted on being referred, and discounted his wife's efforts to help him. He would take no responsibility for helping himself ('Why don't you . . . yes, but').

Mr Braden p. 64
A patient who insisted that everyone else should try to make his life more comfortable because he had been born with such 'terrible nerves', though he would do nothing himself to improve things ('Wooden Leg').

Mrs Corrigan p. 65
A woman who defended her self-centred behaviour by using the jargon she had learned in many psychiatric clinics. The conditions from which she claimed to suffer exonerated her from blame ('Psychiatry').

Mr & Mrs Dunstable p. 65
A wife who complained that her husband was giving her no support at a time of crisis. He defended his irritable reactions on the grounds that she always ignored his opinions and pushed him around; she insisted that she could not cope properly because she always had to make all the decisions. Each could blame the other when things went wrong, so neither felt any need to change ('See what you made me do'/'Harried').

Mrs Emonds p. 67
A woman who surprised the doctor by behaving in a rational Adult way when she thought that her breast cancer was spreading. He was more accustomed to Childish reactions in such circumstances.

Mrs Farquhar p. 67
A patient who was objective and Adult about her repeated failure to lose weight and who asked to be allowed to be treated like a child by the doctor.

Mrs Grantly p. 67
A woman who blamed her nervous dyspepsia on the fact that the house next door had been bought by Indians. She had no rational basis for her anxieties, which were the judgmental responses of her Parent.

Mr & Mrs Hildren p. 68
A couple whose little daughter cried at night. They wanted sympathy from the doctor, and medication for the child. They were not interested in his Adult professional opinion—only in support from his Parent.

Mrs Ives p. 69
A woman who was galvanised into dieting when the doctor made a remark that was ostensibly addressed by his Adult to hers, but which was effective because it was heard by her Child.

CHAPTER 9—PLAYING GAMES WITH THE DOCTOR

Mrs Ackroyd p. 70
A woman whose requests for night-calls were bound to annoy her doctors but who professed surprise when one of them erupted in anger ('Kick me').

Miss Ballard p. 71
A woman who consulted any of the practice partners when she had a new complaint, but who always went to one particular doctor for follow-up. He was the one she could most easily manipulate into doing things for her because he needed to be seen as helpful regardless of the circumstances ('I'm only trying to help'/'Let's you and him fight').

Mrs Churchill p. 73
An old lady who wanted to take to her bed and tried to get the doctor's agreement by using flattery and 'Wooden Leg'. She was stung by his scornful reaction and made herself mobile again 'just to show him'.

CHAPTER 10—SCRIPTS

Mr Appleyard p. 78
A man whose Script called for him to work himself to the point of breakdown before he was allowed to slow down. He needed a Permission that was powerful enough to let him slow down *before* he had his coronary.

CHAPTER 11—HAPPY AND UNHAPPY FAMILIES

Mrs Arliss p. 80
A woman who encouraged her doctor to take on many of the responsibilities that properly belonged to her husband—who soon found himself another woman.

Mr & Mrs Box p. 81
A couple whose marital problems were signalled by the conditions they presented separately to the doctor. Each precluded him from considering their relationship and left him unable to help.

Mrs Candless p. 81
Instead of encouraging this woman's attempts to cope with her baby the doctor demonstrated her incompetence in front of her husband. The family changed doctors.

Mr & Mrs Derby p. 82
A couple who were exhausted by trying to deal with their fractious baby in the strict and inflexible way they had learned from their parents. Being given permission to respond more spontaneously brought them great relief.

Mrs Everly p. 83
A woman who felt anxious and guilty when her children picked up minor respiratory infections. She was worried about her own adequacy and mental stability because her sister had been admitted to a mental hospital.

Mrs Forrester p. 83
A woman who became very anxious whenever her second child was unwell, though she had not been like that with her first. She had tried to abort her second pregnancy.

Mrs Glazier p. 83
A patient so cowed by her mother that she could not cope with her own spirited daughter. She tried to hide her anger and was dismayed by her weakness.

Mrs Harlan p. 83
A woman who was permissive with her children because she had been brought up very strictly. This was a deliberate policy, but she was still left with expectations of her children that were rather rigid.

Mrs Idle p. 84
A woman who nagged her husband and was too tense to enjoy sex. She had always believed that her father thought she was horrid.

Victor Jobling p. 84
A boy whose mother had been so domineering that he was frightened of women and thought that he must therefore be homosexual.

Kenneth Kent p. 84
A neglected boy who turned to clowning to command attention. He became the family scapegoat, allowing his younger siblings to grow up more normally; this served to emphasise his own disturbed behaviour.

Mrs Law p. 85
A woman whose emotional outbursts made her family regard her as a problem. The doctor saw that she had been manoeuvred into being the 'ill' member by a more seriously disturbed husband who was diverting attention on to her that he could not have tolerated himself.

Mrs Morris p. 85
A woman who could not behave lovingly with her baby. She could think of no way to control him other than giving him sedatives which she sought from the doctor.

Mrs Narovic p. 86
A patient who was very distressed by her daughter's refusal to eat properly. When the doctor got her to talk about her war-time experiences in front of her daughter, the family relationship improved.

The Ormond family p. 87
The parents complained of their 9-year-old son's behaviour but had always doubted their ability to cope with him. He was frightened that he was uncontrollable. The doctor helped the parents to be properly firm and the whole family became happier.

Mrs Pitt p. 88
A woman with abdominal pains which semed to be connected with imminent renal investigations, but which were in fact a reaction to her husband's being charged with indecent exposure.

Mr Quale p. 88
A man with a proven duodenal ulcer whose symptoms occurred in sympathy with his wife's pregnancy symptoms—the Couvade syndrome.

The Roe family p. 89
A complex story involving several generations of two families. In Basil Roe's family the women were all-powerful, while his wife had been brought up to believe that women should be submissive. The patient who presented was not the one most ill; there were several instances of invitations to treat the 'absent' patient; and more members of the families consulted the doctor than he could cope with.

CHAPTER 12—HEALTH BREAKING THROUGH

Susan Anderson p. 94
A girl, exploited by both her boy-friend and her employer, who presented with symptoms of tension. She was helped by the idea that she was not ill but experiencing the stress of beginning to assert her own identity.

Mrs Burns p. 95
A woman whose two previous marriages had taught her that close relationships were bound to end in pain and who had been taking hypnotics for many years to subdue her natural feelings. When the doctor withdrew her tablets she fell in love with him because this seemed safe from consequences, but with his support she was able to risk finding a man from the real world.

CHAPTER 13—ANXIETY

Mrs Allen p. 98
A woman under much strain when her marriage broke down and she was developing a new relationship. She failed to make some important decisions, probably because she was taking tranquillisers.

Mrs Bell p. 99
A woman who could not face either having a baby or terminating her pregnancy, and tried to kill herself (avoidance–avoidance conflict).

Mrs Cullen p. 100
A woman who exhibited anxiety when she had to choose between two long-desired goals—a holiday or a new Council flat (approach–approach conflict).

Mr Doyle p. 101
A conscientious worker offered promotion at work, with better pay, who was frightened he could not cope with the responsibility but scared he would lose his job if he did not take it (approach–avoidance conflict).

Mrs Earle p. 102
A woman who was worried about her daughter's marriage and her grandson's health but who was frightened of interfering. She suffered a series of approach–avoidance conflicts.

Mrs France p. 102
A woman who presented symptoms of anxiety which she always connected with current events. She persistently repressed feelings about much more important factors in her life, perhaps to defend herself against depression.

Miss George p. 104
An agoraphobic patient who was treated by desensitisation, illustrating the ideas of negative and positive reinforcement postulated by learning theory.

Mr Haynes p. 105
A patient whose anxiety seemed to be a personality trait. Dealing with current exacerbations never brought him more than temporary relief.

CHAPTER 14—CHILDREN

John Astley p. 108
A 7-year-old boy with recurrent abdominal pain who was clearly disturbed by the relationship between his divorced parents. The doctor chose to treat him rather than his parents and the pains disappeared.

Gillian Ball p. 109
A 5-year-old girl who started wetting the bed when she went to school. She had to be kept off school when she was feverish in case she had a u.t.i., even though this probably delayed her adjustment.

Tom Camberley p. 110
A 1-year-old who was referred directly to a surgeon by a clinic doctor who could not find one of the boy's testes. The mother was badly upset and the general practitioner was annoyed because he knew that there was nothing wrong.

Colin Dilley p. 110
A 9-year-old boy who was brought by his mother because he could not sit still. He was quite seriously disturbed, and well-meaning efforts by everyone in the past to make allowances for him had done more harm than good.

Nigel Eggleton p. 112
A baby whose mother thought he needed circumcising because his foreskin would not retract fully. The problem was 'liquidated' with an explanation of why operation was unnecessary.

Melissa Finch p. 112
A little girl whose mother thought that her health was poor because she had recurrent colds. When this problem was 'liquidated' the doctor discovered that events in the pregnancy had convinced Mrs Finch that the baby would be abnormal in some way.

Ms Green & her baby p. 113
The doctor tried to redefine the cause of the baby's fretfulness as the parental relationship rather than illness, and to manage the situation accordingly.

Jimmy Hoadley p. 114
An 11-year-old albino with an over-protective mother. His secondary problems vanished when the doctor was able to help her relax.

Miss Isaac & her daughter p. 115
A family who were being seen by a bewildering variety of professionals though not by the general practitioner. No one was taking overall responsibility though each was doing his best—a classic instance of the 'collusion of anonymity', which the mother was in fact encouraging.

CHAPTER 15—THE ELDERLY

Mrs Andrews p. 117
An old lady who had declined the many services for which her general practitioner had referred her; even lying in a mess of faeces and urine she was still fiercely proud.

Mrs Barron p. 118
A very elderly lady with a coryza who took to her bed to force her daughter to come back home.

Mr & Mrs Collins p. 120
A well-adjusted couple where the husband responded to his disabilities in an active and constructive way while his wife was happy to be dependent on him. Moving to be near their son would have destroyed the reasonably stable situation they had created for themselves.

Mrs Davis p. 122
An old lady whose demented and paranoid behaviour was caused by the drugs she was taking: the purposes of two medicines had been confused.

Mrs Edge p. 123
A woman whose doctor got to know her while he was weaning her off unnecessary anti-hypertensive treatment. She had a long-standing depression which might have been diagnosed and possibly cured many years earlier.

CHAPTER 16—A MATTER OF CONFIDENCE

Mrs Argyle & her son p. 125
Mrs Argyle told the doctor that she had given her son a spurious alibi, but the doctor

was not bound to tell the police this because the evidence about the boy was second-hand. When the boy himself confirmed his guilt the situation was different and the doctor could not logically defend inaction on the grounds that the crime was not a serious one.

Mr Billings p. 127
A young man who said he was depressed, though in fact he was scared because he was being charged with stealing. He was not at all upset when the doctor pointed out that both the charge and the reaction were justifiable.

Mrs Campbell p. 128
A woman who tried to enlist the doctor's sympathy by lying about her husband's behaviour and who manipulated her son so that he believed the stories too. The doctor fell into the trap of believing the accusations and also erred in revealing to the son what his mother had said.

CHAPTER 17—TREATING THE CAUSE

Mrs Ashworth p. 131
A patient whose depression was accurately but over-hastily diagnosed. She interpreted his haste in terms of her feelings of worthlessness and failed to take the treatment.

Mrs Berwick p. 132
A woman with symptoms that were probably due to an upset in her new marriage. The doctor chose to treat her at a physical level because he did not know enough about her to warrant interfering with the development of the marital relationship.